Frailty in Aging

Interdisciplinary Topics in Gerontology and Geriatrics

Vol. 41

Series Editor

Tamas Fulop Sherbrooke, Que.

Frailty in Aging

Biological, Clinical and Social Implications

Volume Editors

Olga Theou Halifax, N.S.

Kenneth Rockwood Halifax, N.S.

22 figures and 6 tables, 2015

KARGER Basel · Freiburg · Paris · London · New York · Chennai · New Delhi · Bangkok · Beijing · Shanghai · Tokyo · Kuala Lumpur · Singapore · Sydney

Dr. Olga Theou
Center for Health Care of the Elderly
Nova Scotia Health Authority
5955 Veterans' Memorial Lane, Suite 1313
Halifax, NS B3H 2E1
Canada

Prof. Kenneth Rockwood
Centre for Health Care of the Elderly
Nova Scotia Health Authority
5955 Veterans' Memorial Lane, Suite 1421
Halifax, NS B3H 2E1
Canada

Library of Congress Cataloging-in-Publication Data

Frailty in aging : biological, clinical, and social implications / volume editors, Olga Theou, Kenneth Rockwood.
p. ; cm. -- (Interdisciplinary topics in gerontology and geriatrics, ISSN 2297-3508 ; vol. 41)
Includes bibliographical references and index.
ISBN 978-3-318-05456-9 (hard cover : alk. paper) -- ISBN (invalid) 978-3-318-05457-6 (electronic version)
I. Theou, Olga, editor. II. Rockwood, Kenneth, editor. III. Series: Interdisciplinary topics in gerontology ; 41. 2297-3508
[DNLM: 1. Frail Elderly. W1 IN679 v.41 2015 / WT 104]
HV1451
362.6--dc23

2015016199

Bibliographic Indices. This publication is listed in bibliographic services, including Current Contents® and PubMed/MEDLINE.

www.karger.com
Printed in Germany on acid-free and non-aging paper (ISO 9706) by Kraft Druck, Ettlingen
ISSN 2297–3508
e-ISSN 2297–3486
ISBN 978–3–318–05456–9
e-ISBN 978–3–318–05457–6

KARGER 125 YEARS

Contents

Introduction

People today generally live longer and healthier lives than at any other point in history. This 'demographic transition' and its associated 'epidemiological transition' of changing disease patterns affect the global population. Due to low birth and mortality rates, national populations are aging at a rapidly increasing rate. Almost one in seven Canadians and one in every five Europeans is older than 65. Furthermore, the number of older adults is expected to double by 2036, and those older than 80 years are the fastest growing segment of the population. This is particularly important because it is amongst those aged 80+ years that health care use becomes especially disproportionate, with people aged 80+ composing little more than 2% of the population, but consuming 20% of adult, nonobstetrical hospital days.

To understand the impact of these well-known trends, we need to consider the achievements in medical technology and the increase in age-associated, noncommunicable diseases. As a consequence, many more people are able to tolerate more health deficits without dying. In Canada, 91% of older adults have at least one chronic condition, 50% have five or more, and 40% live with a disability. Canadian older adults account for 45% of all health care expenditures, and estimates from elsewhere show comparable results. This would be unproblematic if older adults received care that justified the expenditures, but that appears to not always be the case. Indeed, the growing number of adults with multiple, interacting medical and social problems is proving to be an important challenge in providing quality health care. Specifically, we need health systems that are appropriate to the needs of older adults, especially those who have more than one acute illness and who come from social environments that might not fully support their post-acute care needs.

Not every older adult has multiple problems, and in a haste to correct this perception, there can be a tendency to go too far in the other direction, as though no older adults have special needs. As one notorious health-planning paper put it, 'the aging of the population matters less than you think'. However, variability in health status is an important phenomenon that becomes more important with age. Some older adults remain healthy even to a very old age, whereas other will experience multiple health problems from middle age [1, 2]. In geriatric medicine, the concept of frailty has been introduced to capture this variability in the rate of aging. This term is also used by demographers and actuaries to denote a fixed factor that is associated with a shortened lifespan. In contrast, geriatricians see the frailty state as changing over the life course. The question of whether people have a lifelong predisposition to what geriatricians call frailty has not been resolved.

Frailty is noncontroversially understood as the concept of increased vulnerability to adverse outcomes among people of the same chronological age. Adverse outcomes associated with frailty include falls, cognitive impairment, disability, hospitalization, institutionalization, and death [3–7]. Frailty arises from a multisystem compromising the body's ability to repair [8], which is essential in aging organisms that face a variety of potentially damaging insults. Much of the damage arises as the inevitable result of metabolism – for example in oxidative stress. The environment clearly impacts how much damage arises and how damage can be repaired over time. However, at present, we have only limited evidence about the association between cellular aging markers and frailty [9, 10].

Frailty represents an important challenge for aging populations. Pragmatically, at some point, the number of things that people have wrong with them becomes more important than the exact nature of what they have wrong with them, at least with respect to what they need and how their medical care is best administered. This is so even though, for individuals, it will always be important to know what exactly is wrong. Still, at some point, the complexity of needs in frail individuals means that knowing exactly what is wrong is best achieved in ways that allow complexity to be embraced. This approach of embracing complexity by looking at measures of whole-system function (cognition, mobility, balance, independence in daily activities) is in contrast to the problem list method, a long and widely used approach in medicine. Using the problem list approach, each problem present in an individual is enumerated and addressed, typically one problem at a time. However, when people are frail and have many things wrong with them, the better approach is to look for problems that indicate whole-system difficulty and to address those at the system level. For example, mobility impairment will always be important no matter what the cause; consequently, focusing on mobilizing patients will always be important. This holds true even in cases (such as tibial plateau fractures) in which early mobilization will need to be restricted. Likewise, being able to diagnose mobility impairment in the absence of focal neurological or musculoskeletal problems is essential. For example, weakness is commonly seen in hyponatremic patients, even if the causal chain between having low serum sodium and spending most time in bed is elaborate. Frailty seems to be a good lens through which to refract multimorbidity, dependence, disability and motor slowing (with or without impaired balance or frank disability). Assessing frailty can be done either at the screening level or by a comprehensive geriatric assessment. Given its pervasive impact on health and the outcomes of health care, it has been proposed that frailty should always be considered when treating the older patient [11]. To achieve this, we need tools with sound psychometric properties to assess frailty in clinical settings [12].

Even so, there is still heated debate over how to achieve consensus regarding the best definition of frailty for clinical uses [13].

Even though much has been done to advance our understanding of frailty, it is a concept full of 'known unknowns', such as the mechanisms leading to frailty and the management of frailty [14]. In order to examine these 'known unknowns' and to start considering the 'unknown unknowns', the new science of understanding and managing frailty requires an appropriate framing of the problem. This book aims to consider these and related questions. How can we recognize frailty? How does an understanding of frailty inform our understanding of the aging process? What are its more general implications for health care systems and society? To achieve these goals, we asked the authors to focus on the key points that are known in their area and then to put this information into the framework of frailty as a vulnerability state. We then asked for an arbitrary restriction of the number of references and for them to provide some key unanswered questions in their area. In this way, we hope that this book will be useful in summarizing what we now know and where we will go with these inquiries.

In the first section of the book, 'The biology of frailty', we begin by trying to understand the link between cellular deficit accumulation and the manifestation of microscopic/clinically visible deficits. We discuss how frailty might arise through the biological processes of metabolism, aging, and the accumulation of these subcellular deficits. In Chapter 2, we describe recent advances in animal models of deficit accumulation and the assessment of frailty in animals. In Chapter 3, we examine the role of faulty repair mechanisms that allow damage to accumulate, giving rise to frailty. These mechanisms include oxidative stress with metabolism, DNA repair, inflammation, and the aging of the immune system – 'immunosenescence'. What is known regarding sex differences in frailty is laid out in Chapter 4. Concluding the first section, Chapter 5 considers the relationship between aging, frailty, and the microbiome.

In the second section, 'Evaluation and management of frailty', we begin by discussing how frailty is conceptualized and operationalized based on various approaches, including the two most common approaches – the frailty phenotype and the accumulation of deficits. In Chapter 8, we outline the importance and usefulness of identifying frailty early in primary care settings and further how frailty might be screened for and prevented. Chapter 9 describes how hospital-based care can be best organized to the benefit of frail older adults, who often present with multiple, interacting medical and social problems. Chapter 10 underscores how mobility can be an important marker of frailty and how frailty might be assessed by tracking mobility alone. Subsequently, we will describe the benefits of interprofessional collaborative practice for the care of frail older adults in Chapter 11, and we review the challenges and opportunities for rehabilitation in frail patients, who often experience rapid deconditioning, in Chapter 12. End-of-life care for frail older patients and how to best synthesize palliative and therapeutic care are each considered in Chapter 13.

The 'Social aspects of frailty' section begins by describing how the assessment of frailty can usefully inform the further organization of clinical care. Ethical and legal implications of frailty are discussed in Chapter 15, and the relationship between frailty, social vulnerability, and adverse outcomes is considered in Chapter 16.

Kenneth Rockwood, Halifax, N.S.
Olga Theou, Halifax, N.S.

References

1 Mitnitski A, Song X, Rockwood K: Improvement and decline in health status from late middle age: modeling age-related changes in deficit accumulation. Exp Gerontol 2007;42:1109–1115.

2 Romero-Ortuno R, O'Shea D: Fitness and frailty: opposite ends of a challenging continuum! Will the end of age discrimination make frailty assessments an imperative? Age Ageing 2013;42:270–280.

3 Fried LP, Tangen CM, Walston J, et al: Frailty in older adults: evidence for a phenotype. J Gerontol A Biol Sci Med Sci 2001;56:M146–M156.

4 Mitnitski AB, Mogilner AJ, Rockwood K: Accumulation of deficits as a proxy measure of aging. ScientificWorldJournal 2001;1:323–336.

5 Bergman H, Béland F, Karunanathan S, et al: Developing a working framework for understanding frailty. Gérontologie et Société 2004;109:15–29.

6 Fulop T, Larbi A, Witkowski JM, et al: Aging, frailty and age-related diseases. Biogerontology 2010; 11:547–563.

7 Woo J, Leung J, Morley JE: Comparison of frailty indicators based on clinical phenotype and the multiple deficit approach in predicting mortality and physical limitation. J Am Geriatr Soc 2012;60: 1478–1486.

8 Clegg A, Young J, Iliffe S, et al: Frailty in elderly people. Lancet 2013;381:752–762.

9 Collerton J, Martin-Ruiz C, Davies K, et al: Frailty and the role of inflammation, immunosenescence and cellular ageing in the very old: cross-sectional findings from the Newcastle 85+ Study. Mech Ageing Dev 2012;133:456–466.

10 Claesson MJ, Jeffery IB, Conde S, et al: Gut microbiota composition correlates with diet and health in the elderly. Nature 2012;488:178–184.

11 Theou O, Rockwood K: Should frailty status always be considered when treating the elderly patient? Aging Health 2012;8:261–271.

12 de Vries NM, Staal JB, van Ravensberg CD, et al: Outcome instruments to measure frailty: a systematic review. Ageing Res Rev 2011;10:104–114.

13 Rodriguez-Manas L, Feart C, Mann G, et al: Searching for an operational definition of frailty: a Delphi method based consensus statement. the frailty operative definition-consensus conference project. J Gerontol A Biol Sci Med Sci 2012;68:62–67.

14 Hubbard RE, Theou O: Frailty: enhancing the known knowns. Age Ageing 2012;41:574–575.

Theou O, Rockwood K (eds): Frailty in Aging. Biological, Clinical and Social Implications.
Interdiscipl Top Gerontol Geriatr. Basel, Karger, 2015, vol 41, pp 1–14 (DOI: 10.1159/000381127)

Frailty: Scaling from Cellular Deficit Accumulation?

Kenneth Rockwood[a–c, e, g] • Arnold Mitnitski[c] • Susan E. Howlett[a, c, d, f, h]

Divisions of [a]Geriatric Medicine and [b]Neurology, Department of Medicine, and Departments of [c]Medicine and [d]Pharmacology, Dalhousie University, Halifax, N.S., Canada; Departments of [e]Geriatric Medicine and [f]Physiology, and Institutes of [g]Brain, Behaviour and Neurosciences, and [h]Cardiovascular Sciences, University of Manchester, Manchester, UK

Abstract

Cells age in association with deficit accumulation via mechanisms that are far from fully defined. Even so, how deficits might scale up from the subcellular level to give rise to clinically evident age-related changes can be investigated. This 'scaling problem' can be viewed either as a series of little-related events that reflect discrete processes – such as the development of particular diseases – or as a stochastic process with orderly progression at the systems level, regardless of which diseases are present. Some recent evidence favors the latter hypothesis, but determining the best approach to study how deficits scale remains a key goal for understanding aging. In consequence, approaching the problem of frailty as one of the scaling of subcellular deficits has implications for understanding aging. Considering the cumulative effects of many small deficits appears to allow for the observation of important aspects of the behavior of systems that are close to failure. Mathematical modeling offers useful possibilities in clarifying the extent to which different clinical scales measure different phenomena. Even so, to be useful, mathematical modelling must be clinically coherent in addition to mathematically sound. In this regard, queuing appears to offer some potential for investigating how deficits originate and accumulate.

Frailty and Age-Related Deficit Accumulation

With age, the risk of death accelerates. Still, not everyone at the same age has the same risk of death. People who are at an increased risk of death compared to others of the same age are said to be *frail*. Considered in this way – as a risk state – the basis of frailty appears to be related to the number of things that people have wrong with them.

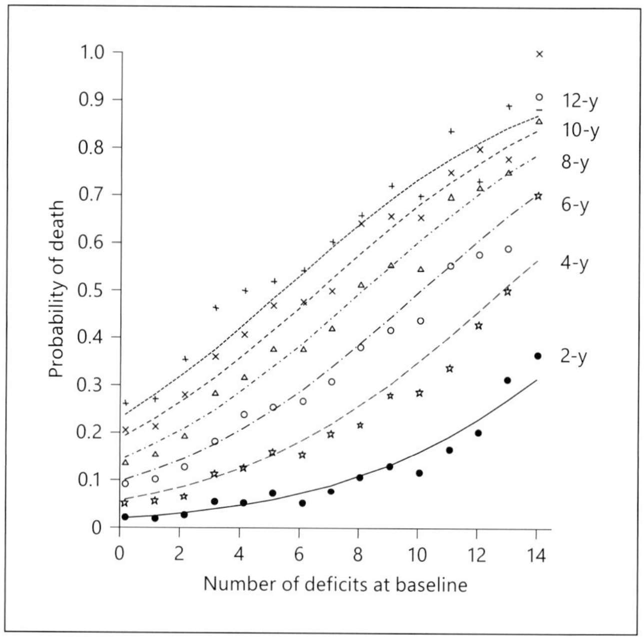

Fig. 1. Mortality in relation to deficit accumulation. Mortality over 12 years according to the number of deficits at baseline. The deficit accumulation approach allows frailty to be stratified; the higher the number of deficits, the higher the risk of a range of adverse outcomes.

In the tradition of understanding frailty as a risk state that is operationalized through deficit accumulation, we call these 'things wrong' *health deficits*. This conception makes a beguiling argument: frailty was proposed as way to describe greater vulnerability of some people to adverse health outcomes compared with others. (Its counterpart – a lower risk of adverse health outcomes, is generally understood as fitness.) Just as not every person of the same age has the same risk of death, not everyone at the same age has the same number of deficits. So, the argument follows that it is the people with the greater number of deficits who appear to be at the greatest risk of death, other things being equal. (As would also be expected, those with the fewest things wrong have the lowest risk of death.) This hypothesis generally seems to be true [1] (fig. 1). This argument also holds for the 'frailty phenotype' approach, in which mortality increases as individuals accumulate the five deficits specified in that definition of frailty (weakness, slowness, weight loss, exhaustion, and reduced activity); it even holds for a random sampling of deficits, such that if any 5, or 10 or 15 deficits are specified, the more of these that people have, the greater their risk of death [2].

This evidence seems to reflect that aging itself can be understood as the accumulation of deficits from subcellular processes to tissues to organs that manifest as clinical changes [3]. As a consequence, a further argument that unites aging, deficit accumulation and frailty is that cellular and molecular deficits scale up to produce clinically detectable deficits [4]. If so, then cellular deficit accumulation should be associated with frailty. Recent preliminary evidence, discussed below, seems to support this argument, too [5]. Even so, questions remain about whether the whole story of cellular deficit accumulation ultimately leading to frailty – considered as a form of accelerated aging – is plausible and what this understanding might add if it were the case. Those questions form the basis for this chapter.

Cellular Events in Aging

Cellular aging arises when *damage* is unrepaired or is not removed, giving rise to *deficits*. How damage arises is an area of contention. For a long time, it was understood that damage could arise endogenously (e.g. reactive oxygen species produced as by-products of metabolism) or exogenously (e.g. radiation, hypothermia, or hypoxemia). The inevitability of damage means that viability requires a variety of repair mechanisms, including an elaborate DNA repair response [6]. Chromosomal damage induces telomerase activity, and autophagy exemplifies a damage removal mechanism. As discussed below, these mechanisms and several others were the subject of a 2013 paper in Cell, entitled 'The Hallmarks of Aging' [7].

It now seems that endogenous damage also occurs as a result of specific metabolic pathways, notably the mechanistic target of rapamycin (mTOR) pathway. mTOR is a serine/threonine protein kinase that interacts with specific adaptor proteins to form two structurally and biologically distinct complexes, mTOR complex 1 (mTORC1) and mTOR complex 2 [8]. mTORC1 regulates processes including cell growth and proliferation, protein synthesis, autophagy and metabolism, whereas mTOR complex 2 is thought to be involved in cytoskeletal organization and cell survival [8, 9]. The mTOR pathway is dysregulated in a variety of disease states including cardiovascular disease and cancer [8]. Interestingly, the inhibition of mTORC1 has been shown to prolong the lifespan of mice [9], and the inhibition of so-called mTOR hyperactivation has been implicated in cellular aging, with some evidence that its inhibition has favorable effects on stem cells [10]. If so, then an important consequence is that aging in this sense becomes more like disease, particularly indicating that aging is potentially susceptible to intervention.

The contemporary understanding of how cellular aging influences tissue function posits an essential role of the phenomenon of cellular senescence, in which dividing cells enter permanent cell cycle arrest. In that state, however, far from being inactive, these cells secrete inflammatory proteins to promote chronic inflammation – so-called 'sterile' inflammation because there is no inciting antigen [11]. These 'senescence-associated secretory phenotype' cells release a variety of factors that might indeed promote not only inflammatory damage but also cancer [11]. Whereas an earlier understanding of cellular senescence posited it as a means by which tumorigenesis could be avoided, it now appears that cellular senescence may in fact give rise to more widespread damage, including cancer. As a consequence, this represents, amongst other things, an important example of how cellular damage might accumulate to give rise to lethal tissue and organ damage, by means of both the accumulation of deficits (the senescent cells) and their damaging effects on nearby – and ultimately distant – cells [12].

A further example of how cellular deficits might give rise to organ dysfunction is seen in the aging brain. Despite substantial and systematic inter- and intra-individual differences, human brain cells accumulate deficits with age. The interpretation of what this means has been re-evaluated in light of attempts to diagnose Alzheimer's disease prior to the presentation of clinically important dementia symptoms. It used to be believed that dementia arose as a consequence of extraneuronal plaques and intracellular tangles. This is now understood to be only part of a more complicated story that is still evolving. The keys to the change in our understanding of the role of plaques and tangles were findings from not only clinic-based necroscopies but also large, prospective, community-based autopsy studies. These studies demonstrate that especially among the very old, many people with normal cognitive function have a considerable burden of neuropathological features that would have enabled the 'definitive' diagnosis of Alzheimer's disease or vascular dementia had clinical dementia been present. In fact, an early, large study reported that no cut-off value of either neuropathological or ischemic lesions discriminated between people with and without dementia [13]. One interpretation of these findings is that scaling from microscopic insults to cognitive dysfunction appears to reflect the total burden of all insults more so than the cumulative burden of any single type of lesion [14].

These findings suggest the need to discriminate structural damage from functional deficits. Even at the cellular level, more damage may make deficits more likely, but deficits are not inevitable. In addition to the evidence from neuropathology, consider the relationship between impaired heart cell structure and function. Although age-dependent changes in cardiomyocytes in and of themselves do not always result in overt cardiac dysfunction, age makes cardiac contractile dysfunction more likely, often through impaired calcium homeostasis [15]. Still, before calcium homeostasis becomes compromised, other changes are evident. At the cellular level, aberrant proteins accumulate, defective mitochondria are seen and mitochondrial function is reduced [16, 17]. In postmitotic cells, the failure of damage removal is key, and lipofuscin (proteinaceous debris consisting of a nondegradable intralysosomal substance made up of cross-linked proteins) is evident [16]. At the tissue level, myocytes are progressively lost, and surviving myocytes undergo hypertrophy, especially in older males, as shown in both human and animal studies [18].

To determine how frailty might relate to cardiomyocyte hypertrophy and dysfunction, we developed a novel frailty index based on deficit accumulation in aging mice [5]. We conducted a cross-sectional study of two groups of mice: a 12-month-old (middle-aged) group and a 30-month-old (aged) group. We found that the aged mice had significantly higher frailty index scores than the younger animals (frailty index = 0.43 ± 0.03 vs. 0.08 ± 0.02; $p < 0.001$). Interestingly, the highest frailty index scores were seen for both hypertrophy (fig. 2a, b) and cardiomyocyte contractile dysfunction (fig. 2c, d). This cardiomyocyte contractile dysfunction and hypertrophy is predicted

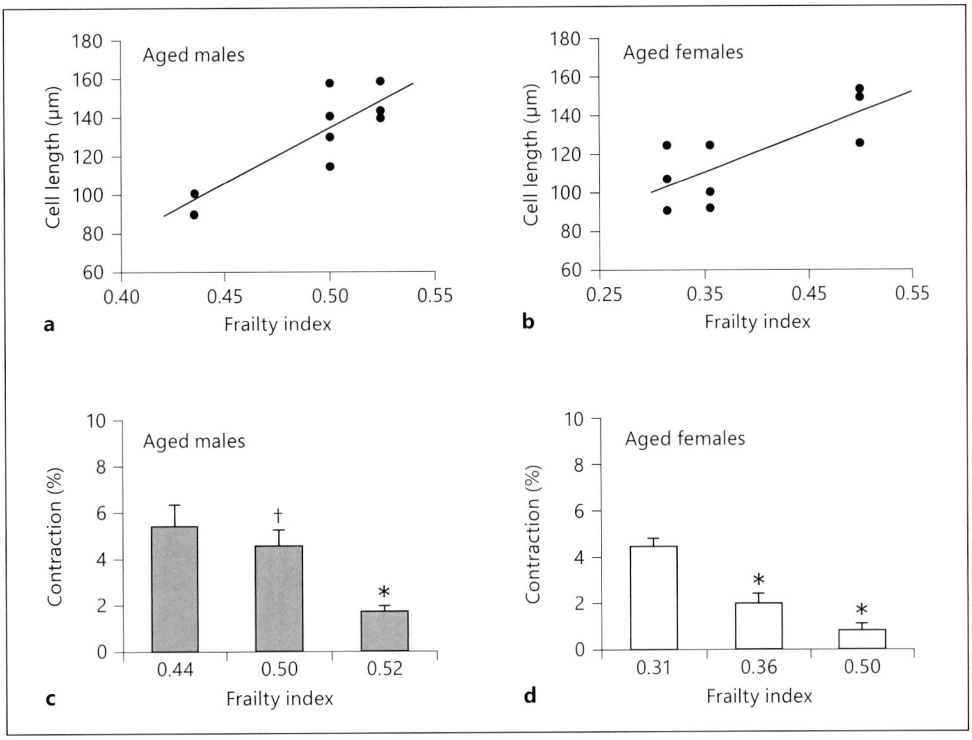

Fig. 2. Relationship between frailty index scores and cardiomyocyte structure and function in a mouse model. **a, b** Cardiomyocyte length increased as the frailty index scores increased in cells from both male mice ($r^2 = 0.76$; $p = 0.001$; $n = 10$ myocytes) and female mice ($r^2 = 0.58$; $p = 0.017$; $n = 9$ myocytes). **c, d** The average (± SEM) amplitude of cardiomyocyte contraction declined as the frailty index scores increased in myocytes from both male and female mice. The cells were paced at 6 Hz; contractions were expressed as fractional shortening (n = 10 and 9 myocytes from aged males and females, respectively). * Denotes a significant difference from the cells from mice with the lowest frailty index; † indicates a significant difference from the cells from mice with the highest frailty index [5].

to result in tissue and organ hypertrophy and contractile dysfunction in vivo, although this hypothesis has yet to be investigated. Our original procedure to measure frailty in aged mice involved specialized equipment and invasive techniques, so this method is not suitable for the longitudinal assessment of frailty [5]. More recently, we have developed a new, noninvasive method to quantify frailty with a frailty index based on the accumulation of clinically apparent deficits in health [19]. Our ongoing studies are using this new clinical frailty index to investigate how cellular deficits in cardiomyocytes of frail mice might scale up to induce overt cardiac dysfunction in the setting of frailty.

In summary, even when cells are damaged, this circumstance need not result in overt changes in organ function if there is compensation for that damage. The nature of this compensation may include the repair or the removal of the damage and may reflect redundancy that allows the damage to be tolerated without any clinical manifestations of illness. Ultimately, however, the accumulation of damage limits the ability to sustain further damage without the expression of disease, leading to what is often termed a loss of physiological reserve. However, this term is controversial in relation to frailty, as it threatens to produce a circular argument. First, if the concept of frailty is meant to operationalize the idea of variable vulnerability to adverse outcomes among people of the same age, then what do we do with the variable vulnerability to adverse outcomes among people who are frail? Is that in any way explained by saying that frail people have varying levels of physiological reserve? The frailty index expresses degrees of frailty (in relation to the degree of deficit accumulation), but what do we say of people with variable outcomes who have similar frailty index scores? Adding the notion of impaired physiological reserve is not helpful here, either. Given that the outcomes (i.e. death or a change in the frailty state/the deficit count) conform to a stochastic process, some degree of variability is to be expected, likely in relation to the degree of damage to which an individual is exposed or to the resources that they can access to repair damage [20]. Each experience (of damage or access to repair) is estimated to some extent by the idea of social vulnerability (see Chapter 16). As discussed below, they can also be modeled by queuing theory.

Additional factors may be important in understanding why the same level of deficit accumulation does not convey the same lethality in all people. More recent studies by our group have investigated the value of a protection index that counts, for example, the positive effects of exercise in addition to the negative effects of a sedentary state [21]. While frailty may define our susceptibility to risk, the rate of damage accumulation must also be considered. These new considerations require revisions of the conceptual basis of deficit accumulation, as described in the next section.

The Origin of Deficit Accumulation

'The Hallmarks of Aging' paper [7] was self-consciously modeled on two other papers in *Cell* entitled the 'Hallmarks of Cancer'. Together, they did much to provide a conceptual focus for research efforts in cancer biology [22]. Even so, these findings were not without their critics. One criticism of special interest to aging research stems from the concern that too narrow a focus was placed on mechanisms of mutations within cells, 'the lowest possible level of organization at which carcinogenesis takes place' [23]. This level of focus comes at the expense of understanding events across cells. In contrast to the somatic mutation theory of cancer, it was proposed that cancer should be seen as a disease of tissues in addition to a disease of cells. In particular, the counterargument notes that cancer metastases require not only malignant cells but also fibroblasts [23]. These fibroblasts operate to give rise to clinical cancer in ways that have received much less attention than individual subcellular mechanisms. According to this argument, understanding how cancer cells and their environment interact is vital to understanding how cancer metastasizes, which requires a focus on events outside the cancer cells; this concept too often gets neglected.

The 'not only cells but also their interactions' critique is compelling to biological gerontologists because, as is often pointed out, the fundamental components of matter do not age [24]. Aging occurs due to the interaction between a variety of components; it is a systems phenomenon. 'The Hallmarks of Aging' authors recognized this. Indeed, 'altered intercellular communication' is presented as one such hallmark, and the mutually reinforcing nature of several other aging hallmarks is seen to reinforce the aging process. As such, we are obliged to understand any given mechanism in the context in which it occurs.

The context, or systems-level behavior, can be captured in general ways and can serve as means of broadly understanding mechanisms. Our group has proposed that in a general way, deficits arise when damage is unremoved or unrepaired [25]. At the level of macroscopic deficits, it appears that the concept of queuing theory offers some useful tools and insights, as discussed below.

Understanding how deficits arise requires an overview of what needs to be explained. With respect to aging, some essential features arise from a consideration of how deficits accumulate. One feature is the substantial individual heterogeneity in the rate at which people accumulate deficits. Similarly, although everyone eventually accumulates deficits, not everyone accumulates the same deficits. In short, there is a strong stochastic influence in how damage accumulates; likewise, the dynamic nature of growth, development and repair is noted as an essential feature of aging, originating from the stochastic nature of the cellular and molecular mechanisms of aging [4].

Our group's stochastic model of the origin of deficit accumulation is based on interactions between two processes: damage occurrence (from environmental stresses, metabolic processes, or even, it must be said, hyperfunctional programs) and damage control and recovery [25]. Both damage and recovery are stochastic – each can arise from many factors that cannot be controlled. Our model is based on queuing theory [26]. The model proposes a formal association between the number of deficits that an individual has accumulated and the length of a queue. In turn, the rate of arrival at the queue reflects the degree of damage that occurs, and the damage repair time represents the recovery time for the individual. In queuing theory, although the equations can be complex, the fundamental principle is governed by what is known as Little's law: $L = \lambda W$, where L is the average length of queue, λ is the average arrival rate and W is the average recovery time. The queue grows longer when many units arrive at it and/or when the processing time is slow. Likewise, deficits accumulate faster in a hazardous environment, when there is a lot of intrinsic damage (arising from particular illnesses, for example) and/or when the recovery time is slow.

This approach seems to hold promise in its application to deficit accumulation. First, queuing theory is used in a variety of applications, particularly communications and computer architecture, in which the information value of the components that make up a system is key. Many aspects of how deficits accumulate are important because of how informative they are about the system as a whole, particularly the degree of vulnerability of the system. Queuing theory offers a useful means of holistically viewing the process of deficit accumulation by taking into account its complex and stochastic nature. Note that the relationships between the macroscopic (average) characteristics of the system are captured by Little's law. These relationships do not depend on the details of particular mechanisms responsible for the formation of the queue (e.g. a single server or a network of servers; stationary or nonstationary arrivals, different priority schedules, etc.). These components, in turn, can be used to model varying environments, intrinsic aging rates and, in particular, systems-level behaviors (such as the length of one queue feeding forward to other queues).

One consequence of evaluating deficit accumulation in this way is that it offers some insight into how recovery potential and deficit accumulation are intertwined. Little's law shows that if the average environmental intensity (λ) is roughly constant over the life span, then W (recovery time) is proportional to N (number of deficits). In short, the increase in the number of deficits reflects the increase in the average recovery time: the more deficits that accumulate, the longer that recovery takes.

The recovery time will clearly increase with age. Because the number of deficits increases by approximately 3% per year [27], we can say that the recovery time increases at the same rate, 3% per year. As a consequence, the number of deficits (in the frailty index) increases threefold from age 65 to age 95 and 10-fold between 20 and 95 years of age [25]. In other words, as the value of the frailty index increases, it takes more time for the individual to recover from any new damage. Relatedly, the increase in the recovery time indicates that deficits would accumulate more rapidly with age even if the intensity of the environmental stresses remained constant throughout the course of life because new damage would take longer to repair, resulting in deficit accumulation over time. Likewise, the average recovery time would continue to increase with age as the number of deficits increased. This index is a means of quantifying what has been termed the 'cycle of frailty', as discussed in Chapter 6 in other contexts.

Frailty at the Organ Level: Variable Organ Dysfunction

The preceding discussion proposes that frailty arises as a consequence of cellular and molecular deficits that accumulate when they are not repaired or removed. This accumulation of microscopic damage may scale up to produce clinically detectable 'macroscopic' deficits at the organ and systems levels. Indeed, there is much evidence that organ system function, at least on average, declines with age. Still, the magnitude of this decline varies substantially, even in individuals who are otherwise well. For example, healthy participants (from 60 to 91 years of age) in the Baltimore Longitudinal Study of Aging (BLSA) showed tremendous variation in peak oxygen consumption during a 400 m walk test [28]. Interestingly, although 17% of these apparently healthy individuals had peak oxygen consumption values that met the disability criterion (<18 ml O_2/kg/min), just as many showed excellent performance, with values >28 ml O_2/kg/min [28]. Analysis of the BLSA cohort also revealed marked heterogeneity in cardiovascular responses to upright bicycle exercise in healthy older adults [29]. While some subjects exhibited impairment in maximal heart rate, end-systolic volume, end-diastolic volume, ejection fraction and cardiac index, others performed at levels equal to or better than younger adults [29]. The effects of age on skeletal muscle quality, mass and strength were strikingly variable in the BLSA cohort [30].

The observation that organ system vulnerability to adverse outcomes varies tremendously, even in healthy older adults, is a further hint of how frailty scales up from the cellular to the organ level. Deficits may accumulate from the organ to the organism as integrated organ function becomes affected (e.g. deficits in mobility). Interestingly, before such organ damage becomes macroscopically visible, it may be detected by laboratory, imaging or electrodiagnostic tests, scaling up from cells to tissues (e.g. from asymptomatic cardiac function to cardiac dysfunction that can be detected by echocardiography). As deficits accumulate at the organ level, they may grow to show symptoms or signs, scaling up to produce overt disease. These observations suggest that what happens at the level of the organ system is not independent of what happens at the cellular level.

Evidence for Scaling in Humans

Whether microscopic deficits scale up to produce organ- and system-level deficits in humans has yet to be extensively investigated. While there are some hints that this may occur [31, 32], there is little direct evidence that microscopic deficits scale up in humans. In fact, frailty index scores are not associated with a decrease in telomere length [33] and are only modestly associated with immune senescence markers, at least when these markers were considered individually [33]. As argued elsewhere, this might reflect that the impact of frailty may be demonstrated less by single values than by the response to a challenge and that the investigation of scaling in humans may require the consideration of more than one deficit or marker. While little is known about how cellular and subcellular deficits might scale up, it seems reasonable that macroscopic deficits must reflect microscopic (or even less detectable) deficits [34]. Recently, our group has reported the first of a series of studies on how abnormal laboratory results can be combined to form a frailty index [35]. In that report, we borrowed from the approach outlined in the development of the initial mouse frailty index [5] and used 21 common laboratory blood tests (e.g. the components of a complete blood count, electrolyte levels, and kidney function to create a laboratory frailty index).

As noted above, the relationship between microscopic deficits, represented by plaques and tangles, in Alzheimer's disease, and disease expression as dementia progresses, might well be related more to the total amount of damage rather than to single processes that underlie how cellular deficits scale up to affect organ systems [3, 13, 14]. Other indirect lines of evidence support the idea that what happens at the microscopic level influences what happens macroscopically and that this scaling occurs in an orderly fashion. Our group has shown that the seemingly patternless changes in deficit accumulation (fig. 3a) are characteristic and depend on the starting state (fig. 3b) [20]. The panels in figure 3b illustrate what happens to the distribution of the deficit count at follow-up in relation to the number of deficits that a person has at baseline. Examples of changes in this distribution are illustrated for baseline/starting states ranging from none (n = 0) to 5 (n = 5). Two changes are evident. First, the areas under the curves diminish as the number of deficits increases, reflecting loss due to mortality. Second, the mode increases by one additional deficit with each iteration; e.g. most people with 1 deficit at baseline have 2 deficits at follow-up, individuals with 3 at baseline have 4 at follow-up, and so on. These changes suggest that, on average, survival declines over time and that survivors accumulate more deficits. Still, despite an average increase in the number of deficits, improvement in health status can occur, as some individuals have fewer deficits at follow-up. Here, we are only concerned with the deficit count; not everyone with the same *number* of deficits has the same *type* of deficits. Even so, despite this inter-individual variability, the overall pattern of change is stable over successive 5 year intervals (fig. 3b). This result is consistent with the idea that on a population basis, it is the number of deficits, not their nature, that is linked to frailty and suggests that any number of shared processes may regulate how damage is repaired or removed.

Mechanisms by Which Frailty Might Emerge from Subcellular Deficits

Studies in an aging animal model have shown that cellular deficits in one organ system (e.g. the heart) correlate with a frailty index calculated from macroscopic deficits in other systems [5]. The mechanism by which frailty elsewhere is associated with frailty in a particular cell type is unclear, although three possibilities suggest themselves. First, subcellular deficits in various organ systems might not be linked in any mechanistic way and might arise because they share the same exposure time. In other words, injury in one system neither protects another system against injury nor predisposes another system to injury, but the more time that elapses, the greater the chance for any system to fail. Second, a common mechanism of injury or incomplete compensatory response might affect more than one cell type [34, 36, 37]. Although there is some evidence for this, as noted, other work has reported no strong relationship, at least when considered individually in cross-sectional data [33]. This could occur if there are many paths to frailty, so that cumulative effects need not have a shared basis or mechanism. In support of this concept, genome-wide association studies in humans have shown that low-significance longevity alleles accumulate to affect survival [32].

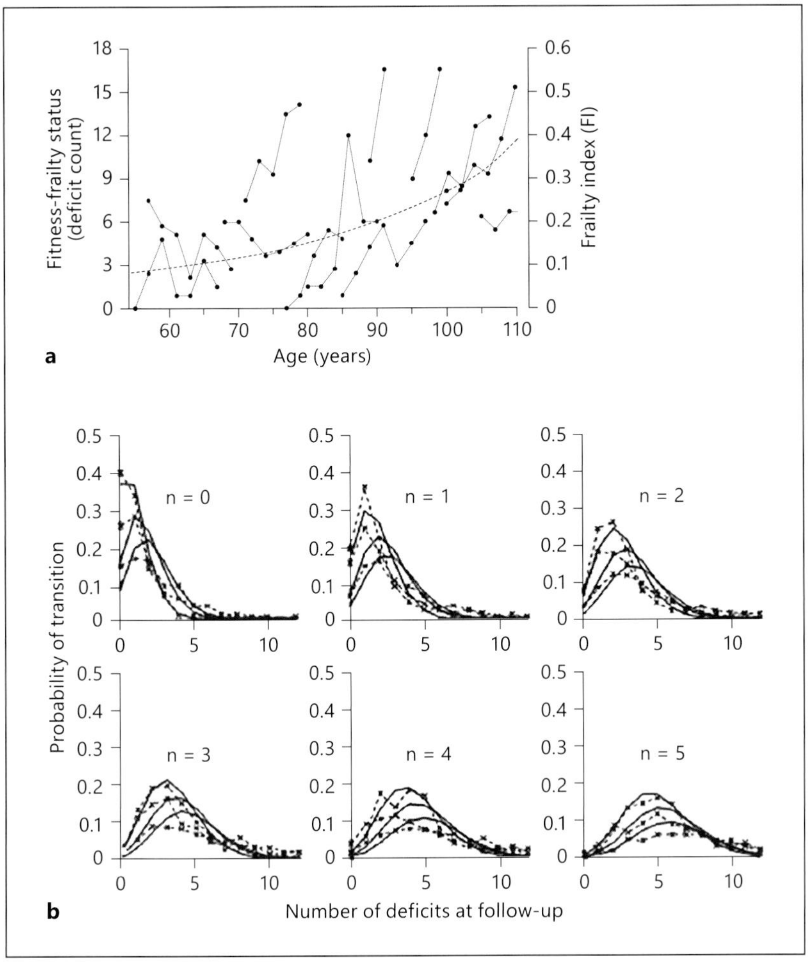

Fig. 3. The distribution of the frailty index characteristically changes in relation to the number of deficits at baseline. **a** Individual trajectories of the number of deficits in successive waves of the National Population Health Survey in relation to age. **b** Although the data presented in (**a**) do not seem to conform to a pattern, other than a slow increase in the mean number of deficits (dotted line), they can be well summarized by a Poisson distribution, which captures the output of a stochastic process. The probability that the number of deficits at baseline changes is plotted for each of 5 deficits at baseline. The data shown are from different waves of the National Population Health Survey, each of which shows similar distributions over each successive follow-up period. Regardless of an increase in the number of baseline deficits from none (n = 0) to 5 (n = 5), most people have more deficits at follow-up, although improvement is noted in some individuals. For example, the people who had 2 deficits at baseline most often have 3 deficits (mode) or more at follow-up, but about 15–20% remain at 2 deficits, and a few improve to have only one deficit at follow-up. The tendency toward worsening is strong enough that even with only 3 deficits, almost no one recovers to having 0 deficits after only 2 years. Note that the area under the curve declines as the number of deficits increases, primarily due to mortality. The patterns are consistent between the cycles, even though everyone is 2 years older at the start of each cycle (from Mitnitski et al. [1]).

Third, failure in one system may predispose another system to fail. For example, in a patient with anemia of any cause, the impact on coronary artery disease is likely to be felt sooner than in a patient with a normal red cell count. This almost certainly occurs such that this mechanism serves as a complementary rather than an alternative explanation to other mechanisms. This explanation would readily fit with how deficit accumulation and repair are intertwined, as suggested by the results of the queuing theory analyses.

Conclusions

Individuals who are frail have problems in many organ systems, and these problems can be quantified as a frailty index based on a deficit count. Even so, a high deficit count suggests a relative increase in risk, not an absolute one, as risk can be enhanced by factors such as social vulnerability (see Chapter 16) or be mitigated by other factors including exercise. Macroscopically detectable deficits, even those detected by laboratory or specialized testing, reflect deficits in organ systems. Nonetheless, the line between cellular deficits and clinically detectable deficits will not be straight, as each deficit reflects an unrepaired insult and these insults need not have only one cause. Moreover, cellular deficits that scale up to produce clinical frailty must exist in multiple organ systems [27].

This view of the biology of frailty both offers insights and presents challenges. Animal research offers the chance to learn more about the mechanisms involved in the development of frailty and provides a model system to test new treatments (see Chapter 2). The use of a frailty index based on the accumulation of deficits in organs other than the one being studied can link subcellular and cellular events to events in the whole organism. In humans, a frailty index based on the accumulation of deficits observed on laboratory, imaging and electrodiagnostic tests might likewise serve as a bridge between cellular, tissue and organ damage. Clinical challenges related to deficit scaling include considering how interventions against frailty might offer insights into their mechanisms. Interventions with widespread effects across a variety of insults and intrinsic repair mechanisms need to be evaluated. Exercise is one compelling example.

The notion that widespread age-related deficit accumulation is associated with a variety of late life illnesses (not only dementia but also heart disease [38], osteoporosis and its complications) also has implications for how we understand the epidemiology of late life illness. The epidemiology of disease in old age might well not be the same as the epidemiology of disease in midlife. In short, single risk factors are unlikely to fully explain late life illness; 'adjusting for age' appears to mask systematic variability that quantifying frailty reveals.

Progress in understanding the biology of frailty will require substantial effort and better quantitative models. Approaches that build on everyday clinical experience or the intense study of animals as they age, coupled with feasible quantitative measures and analyses drawing on the mathematics of complexity, seems to be a reasonable approach that is motivating further inquiries by our group.

Sources of Funding

This work was supported by grants from the Canadian Institutes of Health Research (CIHR) to SEH [MOP126018] and to Arnold Mitnitski [MOP25388]. Kenneth Rockwood's frailty work is supported by CIHR grants MOP209888, CCI92216, and MOP115006 and the Fountain Innovation Fund of the Queen Elizabeth II Health Sciences Foundation. He receives career support from the Dalhousie Medical Research Foundation as the Kathryn Allen Weldon Professor of Alzheimer Research.

References

1 Mitnitski A, Song X , Rockwood K: Trajectories of changes over twelve years in the health status of Canadians from late middle age. Exp Gerontol 2012; 47:893–899.

2 Rockwood K, Andrew MK, Mitnitski A: A comparison of two approaches to measuring frailty in elderly people. J Gerontol A Biol Sci Med Sci 2007;62:738–743.

3 Howlett SE, Rockwood K: New horizons in frailty: ageing and the deficit-scaling problem. Age Ageing 2013;42:416–423.

4 Kirkwood TB: Systems biology of ageing and longevity. Philos Trans R Soc Lond B Biol Sci 2011;366:64–70.

5 Parks RJ, Fares E, Macdonald JK, Ernst MC, Sinal CJ, Rockwood K, Howlett SE: A procedure for creating a frailty index based on deficit accumulation in aging mice. J Gerontol A Biol Sci Med Sci 2012;67:217–227.

6 Fortini P, Ferretti C, Dogliotti E: The response to DNA damage during differentiation: pathways and consequences. Mutat Res 2013;743–744:160–168.

7 López-Otín C, Blasco MA, Partridge L, Serrano M, Kroemer G: The hallmarks of aging. Cell 2013;153: 1194–1217.

8 Sciarretta S, Volpe M, Sadoshima J: Mammalian target of rapamycin signaling in cardiac physiology and disease. Circ Res 2014;114:549–564.

9 Sharp ZD, Curiel TJ, Livi CB: Chronic mechanistic target of rapamycin inhibition: preventing cancer to delay aging, or vice versa? Interdiscip Top Gerontol 2013;38:1–16.

10 Luo Y, Li L, Zou P, Wang J, Shao L, Zhou D, Liu L: Rapamycin enhances long-term hematopoietic reconstitution of ex vivo expanded mouse hematopoietic stem cells by inhibiting senescence. Transplantation 2014;97:20–29.

11 Tchkonia T, Zhu Y, van Deursen J, Campisi J, Kirkland JL: Cellular senescence and the senescent secretory phenotype: therapeutic opportunities. J Clin Invest 2013;123:966–972.

12 Boyette LB, Tuan RS: Adult stem cells and diseases of aging. J Clin Med 2014;3:88–134.

13 Neuropathology Group, Medical Research Council Cognitive Function and Aging Study: Pathological correlates of late-onset dementia in a multicentre, community-based population in England and Wales. Neuropathology Group of the Medical Research Council Cognitive Function and Ageing Study (MRC CFAS). Lancet 2001;357:169–175.

14 Gelber RP, Launer LJ, White LR: The Honolulu-Asia Aging Study: epidemiologic and neuropathologic research on cognitive impairment. Curr Alzheimer Res 2012;9:664–672.

15 Fares E, Howlett SE: Effect of age on cardiac excitation-contraction coupling. Clin Exp Pharmacol Physiol 2010;37:1–7.

16 Sheydina A, Riordon DR, Boheler KR: Molecular mechanisms of cardiomyocyte aging. Clin Sci (Lond) 2011;121:315–329.

17 Kowald A, Dawson, M, Kirkwood, TB: Mitochondrial mutations and ageing: can mitochondrial deletion mutants accumulate via a size based replication advantage? J Theor Biol 2014;340:111–118.

18 Farrell SR, Ross JL, Howlett SE: Sex differences in mechanisms of cardiac excitation-contraction coupling in rat ventricular myocytes. Am J Physiol Heart Circ Physiol 2010;299:H36–H45.

19 Whitehead JC, Hildebrand BA, Sun M, Rockwood MR, Rose RA, Rockwood K, Howlett SE: A clinical frailty index in aging mice: comparisons with frailty index data in humans. J Gerontol A Biol Sci Med Sci 2014;69:621–632.
20 Mitnitski A, Bao L, Rockwood K: Going from bad to worse: a stochastic model of transitions in deficit accumulation, in relation to mortality. Mech Ageing Dev 2006;127:490–493.
21 Wang C, Song X, Mitnitski A, Fang X, Tang Z, Yu P, Rockwood K: Effect of health protective factors on health deficit accumulation and mortality risk in older adults in the Beijing longitudinal study of aging. J Am Geriatr Soc 2014;62:821–828.
22 Hanahan D, Weinberg RA: Hallmarks of cancer: the next generation. Cell 2011;144:646–674.
23 Sonnenschein C, Soto AM: The aging of the 2000 and 2011 Hallmarks of Cancer reviews: a critique. J Biosci 2013;38:651–663.
24 Gavrilov LA, Gavrilova NS: The reliability theory of aging and longevity. J Theor Biol 2001;213:527–545.
25 Mitnitski A, Song X, Rockwood K: Assessing biological aging: the origin of deficit accumulation. Biogerontology 2013;14:709–717.
26 Little, JDC: Little's Law as viewed on its 50th anniversary. Operating Research 2011;59:536–549.
27 Rockwood K, Mitnitski A: Frailty defined by deficit accumulation and geriatric medicine defined by frailty. Clin Geriatr Med 2011;27:17–26.
28 Simonsick EM, Fan E, Fleg JL: Estimating cardiorespiratory fitness in well-functioning older adults: treadmill validation of the long distance corridor walk. J Am Geriatr Soc 2006;54:127–132.
29 Lakatta EG: Age-associated cardiovascular changes in health: impact on cardiovascular disease in older persons. Heart Fail Rev 2002;7:29–49.
30 Moore AZ, Caturegli G, Metter EJ, Makrogiannis S, Resnick SM, Harris TB, Ferrucci L: Difference in muscle quality over the adult life span and biological correlates in the Baltimore Longitudinal Study of Aging. J Am Geriatr Soc 2014;62:230–236.
31 Hubbard RE, Woodhouse KW: Frailty, inflammation and the elderly. Biogerontology 2010;11:635–641.
32 Yashin Al, Wu D, Arbeev KG, Stallard E, Land KC, Ukraintseva SV: How genes influence life span: the biodemography of human survival. Rejuvenation Res 2012;14:374–380.
33 Collerton J, Martin-Ruiz C, Davies K, Hilkens CM, Isaacs J, Kolenda C, Parker C, Dunn M, Catt M, Jagger C, von Zglinicki T, Kirkwood TB: Frailty and the role of inflammation, immunosenescence and cellular ageing in the very old: cross-sectional findings from the Newcastle 85+ Study. Mech Ageing Dev 2012;133:456–466.
34 Moskalev AA, Shaposhnikov MV, Plyusnina EN, Zhavoronkov A, Budovsky A, Yanai H, Fraifeld VE: The role of DNA damage and repair in aging through the prism of Koch-like criteria. Ageing Res Rev 2013;12:661–684.
35 Howlett SE, Rockwood MR, Mitnitski AM, Rockwood K: Standard laboratory tests to identify older adults at increased risk of death. BMC Med 2014;12:171.
36 Bishop NA, Lu T, Yankner BA: Neural mechanisms of ageing and cognitive decline. Nature 2010;464:529–535.
37 Sahin E, DePinho RA: Axis of ageing: telomeres, p53 and mitochondria. Nat Rev Mol Cell Biol 2012;13:397–404.
38 Wallace LM, Theou O, Kirkland SA, Rockwood MR, Davidson KW, Shimbo D, Rockwood K: Accumulation of non-traditional risk factors for coronary heart disease is associated with incident coronary heart disease hospitalization and death. PLoS One 2014;9:e90475.

Prof. Kenneth Rockwood
Centre for Health Care of the Elderly
Capital District Health Authority
1421–5955 Veterans' Memorial Lane, Halifax, NS B3H 2E1 (Canada)
E-Mail Kenneth.Rockwood@dal.ca

Theou O, Rockwood K (eds): Frailty in Aging. Biological, Clinical and Social Implications.
Interdiscipl Top Gerontol Geriatr. Basel, Karger, 2015, vol 41, pp 15–25 (DOI: 10.1159/000381131)

Assessment of Frailty in Animal Models

Susan E. Howlett[a–c]

[a]Department of Pharmacology and [b]Division of Geriatric Medicine, Department of Medicine, Dalhousie University, Halifax, N.S., Canada; [c]Department of Physiology, Institute of Cardiovascular Sciences, University of Manchester, Manchester, UK

Abstract

Animal models have contributed greatly to our understanding of the biology of aging and have been used to test new potential interventions to enhance survival. However, whether these interventions can modify frailty in animals is not yet clear, in part because until recently, frailty had not been considered in animal studies of aging. This review is focused on investigations that have attempted to address the issue of frailty, or aspects of frailty, in animal models, including invertebrate and vertebrate models. Some studies have used skeletal muscle weakness or sarcopenia as a surrogate for frailty in aging animals. Others have used genetically altered mice, in which components of human frailty such as inflammation are enhanced. This review also explores a novel approach to quantify frailty with a 'frailty index' based on deficit accumulation in aging animals. The concept of the frailty index is well established in the clinical literature, but recent work suggests that this approach can also be used to measure frailty in aging animals. The ability to quantify frailty in animals is a major step forward in the effort to understand the biology of frailty and to develop new clinical interventions.

Experience tells us that people age at different rates. Because chronological age does not necessarily reflect biological age, the health status of older adults varies from fit to frail. The concept of frailty, which is a state of increased vulnerability to adverse health outcomes relative to people of the same age, was developed to explain the heterogeneity in clinical outcomes between older patients [1]. Frailty is a major health care problem, as frail individuals have higher mortality and worse outcomes and use more health care services than fit people [2]. Preclinical studies have begun to identify promising new interventions that can increase lifespan and healthspan in animal models. However, whether these interventions can attenuate frailty is not known, in part because until recently, frailty has not been evaluated or quantified in animal models of aging.

This review considers studies that have addressed the issue of frailty, or aspects of frailty, in various animal models, with particular emphasis on studies that have developed an approach to quantify frailty. The majority of these investigations have focused on the assessment of skeletal muscle weakness and sarcopenia in aging animals, as these factors are believed to contribute to frailty in older humans. Other studies have explored genetically manipulated models that have been designed to enhance specific components of human frailty, such as inflammation. This review also highlights a new approach to quantify frailty across many different systems with a 'frailty index' based on deficit accumulation in aging animals. The ability to quantify frailty in animal models is a major advance that should accelerate the effort to translate the basic mechanisms underlying cellular dysfunction in aging into meaningful clinical interventions.

Frailty and Its Measurement

The dictionary definition of the word frailty, from the Latin word *fragilis* (to break), is the condition of being weak or delicate. While there is no internationally agreed upon definition of frailty in the medical literature [3], it is generally understood to represent a state of increased vulnerability to adverse health outcomes for older adults of the same chronological age [3]. Frailty is not caused by aging or chronic disease, as it occurs in younger individuals, is not present in all older adults and occasionally occurs in the absence of specific disease conditions [4]. It is currently thought that frailty develops from the interaction of genetic, cellular, physiological and environmental factors, leading to multisystemic physiological decline [4]. Although its cause is not known, its underlying mechanisms may include genetic variation, cellular senescence, loss of telomeres, mitochondrial damage, increased free radical production and poor DNA repair [4]. The ensuing loss of physiological reserve means that even minor stressors (e.g. urinary tract infection, change in medication, or minor injury) can trigger a domino effect that leads to adverse outcomes, including disability, dependency and death, in frail older adults.

A recent systematic review identified 20 different instruments currently used to measure frailty in the clinical literature [5]. One common approach views frailty as a physical phenotype characterized by weight loss, physical exhaustion, weakness, reduced walking speed and low physical activity; older adults are frail if three or more of these factors are present [6]. Although simple, this approach is limited because it does not grade degrees of frailty, even though a 'pre-frail' state is allowed [5]. Furthermore, this view of frailty as a 'phenotype' is focused solely on physical frailty [5]. An alternative measure, developed by Rockwood et al., is known as a 'frailty index' [7]. A frailty index is created by counting the accumulation of deficits in health across many systems in the body. Deficits measured to construct a frailty index include clinical signs, symptoms, diseases, and laboratory and radiographic abnormalities. The number of deficits a person has is expressed as a ratio of the total number of deficits measured to yield an individual frailty index score between 0 (no deficits) and 1 (all deficits present). Studies in humans have shown that the higher the deficit count (or frailty index), the higher the likelihood of adverse health outcomes, especially if 30 or more deficits are counted [8].

There are several advantages to the frailty index approach. The frailty index measures deficits across different physiological systems, so it is not simply focused on physical frailty [5]. It uses a continuous scoring system, so hypotheses related to the impact of frailty on different outcomes can be tested by measuring changes in the frailty index over time in the same individuals. In large population data sets from different developed countries, several features of frailty are characteristic. For example, deficits accumulate at a rate of 3% per year in older adults, and there is a limit to frailty (a frailty index of 0.67) beyond which individuals no longer survive additional deficits [8]. When the frailty index is used as an explanatory value in a multivariate model (e.g. Cox proportional hazards), the effect of age is typically either minimal or no longer present [8]. Thus, the frailty index predicts adverse outcomes in humans independently of age.

Although the concept of frailty is well established in clinical studies, much less is known about frailty in animals. Recently, some studies have begun to address the issue of frailty in aging and genetically manipulated animal models, often using ideas borrowed from the clinical literature. This approach has led to new insights into the understanding and quantification of frailty in a variety of animal models, as discussed below.

The Evaluation of Frailty in Invertebrates

Studies of the biology of aging have used invertebrate model systems to understand the genetic and molecular bases of the aging process. One established invertebrate model is the fruit fly *Drosophila melanogaster*. The fruit fly is an attractive aging model organism for a number of reasons, including its very short lifespan and the availability of a well-developed set of genetic tools designed to manipulate this model. Recent studies have shown that fasting and drug treatments can alter the survival of *Drosophila* [e.g. 9, 10]. These studies also suggested that such treatments may modify frailty in this model, although they did not specifically measure or quantify frailty [e.g. 9, 10]. In theory, it should be possible to evaluate frailty in *Drosophila*. For example, age-related behavioral declines similar to those found in humans have been well characterized in the *Drosophila* model [11]. These deficits include age-related locomotor impairment and age-dependent changes in memory performance [11]. Although such changes could be considered to reflect aspects of frailty in aging flies, it is not clear that any studies have attempted to use these characteristics to develop a scheme to evaluate frailty in this model.

Another commonly used invertebrate model of aging is the nematode *Caenorhabditis elegans*. As with *Drosophila*, features such as a short lifespan and well-characterized genetics make this organism an attractive model to investigate the biology of aging. Aspects of *C. elegans* behavior, including locomotion and feeding, can be quantified across the lifespan with standardized assays. For example, the worms move freely with sinusoidal movements on a solid surface such as an agar plate, and their movement can be tracked over time [e.g. 12, 13]. In a liquid environment, they swim with a thrashing motion, and the number of body bends per unit time can be quantified [e.g. 12–14]. Their feeding behavior can also be measured according to the frequency of pharyngeal pumps in response to food [e.g. 13, 14]. Based in the notion that locomotor decline plays an important role in the development of frailty in humans, a number of studies have used one or more of these physical activity assays as indicators of frailty in the *C. elegans* model.

An early study by Glenn et al. [12] showed that locomotor deficits are detectible in aging *C. elegans*, even relatively early in the aging process. They showed that this age-dependent loss of movement was linked to a decline in muscle tissue integrity and suggested that these deficits were attributable to 'muscle frailty' [12]. More recent studies have also examined neuromuscular aging in the *C. elegans* model. Iwasa et al. [14] showed that aging was associated with dramatic declines in the frequency of body bends during swimming and of pumping during feeding. They proposed that these assays of locomotor decline are a surrogate measure of frailty that can be used to evaluate the 'healthspan' of *C. elegans* [14]. Mulcahy et al. [13] investigated the neuromuscular junction in *C. elegans* as a model system to explore potential targets for intervention to improve muscle strength in frail older adults. They showed that deficits in swimming and pumping in aging *C. elegans* could be overcome by treatment with an acetylcholinesterase inhibitor combined with a nicotinic agonist to enhance neuromuscular transmission [13]. Together, these observations demonstrate that invertebrate models such as the nematode can be used to model aspects of physical frailty that are observed in aging humans. Furthermore, this model may be useful to evaluate potential treatment strategies for muscle weakness in older adults.

In summary, there is emerging evidence that frailty can be evaluated in commonly used invertebrate models of aging, at least with respect to locomotor deficits and physical frailty. A number of studies have shown that standardized assays, including the assessment of locomotion and feeding, may be useful as indicators of frailty in *C. elegans*. Whether additional behavioral assays could be used to evaluate aspects of frailty beyond physical frailty in this model is not yet known. It is also possible that a similar approach could be useful to explore frailty in other commonly used invertebrate models such as *Drosophila*, although this possibility has yet to be investigated. In the long term, the assessment of frailty in these models may help to identify genes that attenuate frailty and may provide insights into novel treatments for frail older adults.

The Assessment of Frailty in Mammals

Biological Age in Mammalian Models

Although invertebrate models have proven very useful for the study of the biology of aging, the majority of studies in this area have used mammalian models. Rats and mice have been particularly popular, in large part due to the relatively short lifespan (~2.5 years) and ease of genetic manipulation of these models. Although rodent models have contributed a great deal to our understanding of the biology of aging, much less is known about frailty in these models.

While frailty *per se* has not been investigated in rodent models until recently, it has long been appreciated that experimental animals of a similar chronological age may have very different 'biological ages'. For example, an early study by Ingram & Reynolds [15] used a battery of psychomotor tests to evaluate biological age in aging male C57BL/6J mice. They evaluated performance on noninvasive activity tasks, including rotarod (balancing on a rotating rod), grip strength, exploratory behavior and wheel running tasks. The results of their cross-sectional study of 24-month-old mice showed that with the exception of the rotarod task, better performance was associated with a longer lifespan [15]. While this study was not specifically designed to evaluate frailty, these findings do support the concept that a broad-based assessment tool may be a useful measure of overall health or biological age in experimental animals.

Sarcopenia and Frailty in Aging Animals

Studies in humans have often defined frailty in terms of weakness, which is linked to the loss of muscle mass (sarcopenia) that accompanies aging [6]. Based on this view, mammalian models of atrophy, cachexia, and sarcopenia have been proposed for the investigation of the basic mechanisms of frailty [16]. Although relatively few studies have directly explored the link between sarcopenia and frailty in mouse and rat models, several groups have developed new approaches to evaluate neuromuscular health in these models. For example, Weber et al. [17] systematically characterized skeletal muscle aging in pre-clinical mammalian models and compared the results obtained between invasive and noninvasive techniques. They showed that an automated micro-X-ray computed tomography imaging system could be used to accurately quantify changes in muscle mass with aging in both rats and mice [17]. As this system can noninvasively evaluate muscle mass in large numbers of animals, it is ideally suited to evaluate potential therapies for sarcopenia in aging animals. Another interesting development is the introduction of a neuromuscular healthspan scoring system for use on aging mice [18]. This neuromuscular healthspan scoring system provides a unique composite score for each animal from three individual scores obtained from the rotarod test, the grip strength test and the maximal isometric force produced by the isolated extensor digitorum longus muscle [18]. In this way, the mean performance decrement with age can be calculated, and the neuromuscular health of an individual mouse can be compared to that of age-matched animals [18]. The authors suggested that this scale could be used to quantify frailty by setting a cutoff value, below which an animal would be considered as frail [18]. These promising new tools may help to evaluate the success of interventions to treat sarcopenia and may be useful to modify the expression of physical frailty in older adults.

Frailty in Genetically Manipulated Mice

The need for an animal model of frailty has been identified as a key step to translate the understanding of the basic mechanisms of cellular dysfunction in aging into treatments. A 2004 conference directed towards a 'Research Agenda on Frailty in Older Adults' proposed that animal models of frailty should exhibit signs and symptoms of human frailty, such as muscle weakness, inflammation and reduced activity levels [19]. Based on these criteria, Walston et al. took an innovative approach to the evaluation of frailty in mammals. They exploited the availability of genetically manipulated mice to propose a 'frail' mouse model that mimics several aspects of human frailty [20]. They evaluated mice that carry a homozygous deletion of the interleukin (IL)-10 gene (IL-$10^{tm/tm}$) as an animal model of frailty [20]. These mice, which were originally developed as a model of inflammatory bowel disease (IBD), are susceptible to IBD, growth retardation, anemia, and early mortality if they are not raised under specific pathogen-free conditions [21]. These mice do not produce the anti-inflammatory cytokine IL-10 and therefore express elevated levels of pro-inflammatory cytokines [21]. Walston et al. [20] showed that IL-$10^{tm/tm}$ mice exhibited inflammation (increased serum IL-6 levels) and muscle weakness at an earlier age than wild-type controls, consistent with several characteristics of human frailty.

More recent studies of IL-$10^{tm/tm}$ mice by this group have extended these original observations. In addition to increased levels of IL-6, older IL-$10^{tm/tm}$ mice have elevated levels of other pro-inflammatory mediators including IL-1β, TNF-α and IFN-γ, along with an increase in the overall mortality rate, compared to wild-type controls [22]. In vivo measurements have shown that skeletal muscle energy metabolism is depressed in the IL-$10^{tm/tm}$ mouse, and this deficiency may contribute to weakness in this model [23]. Finally, IL-$10^{tm/tm}$ mice have been shown to exhibit signs of cardiovascular dysfunction with aging [24]. IL-$10^{tm/tm}$ mice exhibit age-dependent vascular deficits including elevated blood pressure, stiffened blood vessels and endothelial dysfunction compared to wild-type controls [24]. Deficits in cardiac function, specifically reduced ejection fraction, left ventricular end-systolic dilatation and cardiac hypertrophy, have also been demonstrated on echocardiography [24]. However, whether cardiovascular dysfunction in this model is due to the lack of IL-10, the chronic activation of inflammatory pathways or both has yet to be determined.

The development of the IL-$10^{tm/tm}$ mouse as an animal model of frailty is an important advance in the field of aging research. Recent evidence of weakness, cardiovascular dysfunction and increased mortality suggest that this model not only serves as a model of inflammation but also has features of the multisystemic decline characteristic of human frailty. On the other hand, there are limitations to this approach to the study of frailty in animal models. As noted above, if the animals are not maintained under specific pathogen-free conditions, they will develop IBD, growth retardation and anemia. Thus, the extent to which the IL-10$^{tm/tm}$ mouse mimics natural aging is unclear. Furthermore, although the IL-10$^{tm/tm}$ mouse exhibits aspects of frailty that have been described in people, frailty itself has not been measured or quantified in this model.

Quantification of Frailty with a Frailty Index in Mouse Models of Aging
Howlett et al. have recently published two studies that have taken a novel approach to the evaluation of frailty in mammalian models [25, 26]. Based on the concept that frailty can be measured as deficit accumulation in people [8], they used a 'bedside-to-bench' approach to develop a frailty index for use in a mouse model. In the first study, they selected a large number of health-related variables related to the function of systems that are known to change with age in both human and animal models [25]. These variables provided information about the following: (a) *activity*, including distance moved, velocity of movement and rearing frequency; (b) *hemodynamic status*, including heart rate, systolic and diastolic blood pressure; (c) *body composition*, including body mineral content, percent body fat and percent lean tissue; and (d) *basic metabolism and organ function*, including serum electrolyte levels, hematocrit and urea levels [25]. They measured all 31 variables in two groups of male and female C57BL/6J mice, an adult (12-month-old) group and an aged (30-month-old) group and compared these data with mean reference values for sex-matched adult animals [25]. Values that were 1 standard deviation (SD) above or below the mean reference value received a frailty value of 0.25; 2 SD, 0.5; 3 SD, 0.75; and >4 SD, 1 (the maximal frailty value). Parameters that differed by <1 SD received a frailty value of 0. These values were summed and divided by the total number of parameters measured to yield a frailty index for each animal; a mouse with no deficits would have a score of 0, and an animal with maximal deficits for all applicable parameters would have a score of 1 [25]. The results of this study demonstrated that 12-month-old mice had significantly lower frailty index scores than 30-month-old mice, and this result did not differ between the sexes (fig. 1a).

The results of the study by Parks et al. [25] are exciting because they demonstrate, for the first time, that a frailty index based on the idea of deficit accumulation can be used to quantify frailty in aging mice. Nonetheless, one limitation of this study is that the parameters used to construct the frailty index were measured with specialized equipment (e.g. an open field maze for activity measurement, a tail cuff system for blood pressure measurement, an X-ray scanner to measure body composition, a clinical blood analyzer to assess the serum electrolyte levels, etc.). Furthermore, this frailty index is not suitable for longitudinal studies of frailty in mice due to the invasive nature of some of the techniques employed (e.g. repeated exposure to X-rays and the volume of blood required). These limitations may prevent the use of the frailty index in many research laboratories. To address this issue, Parks et al. [25] showed that a

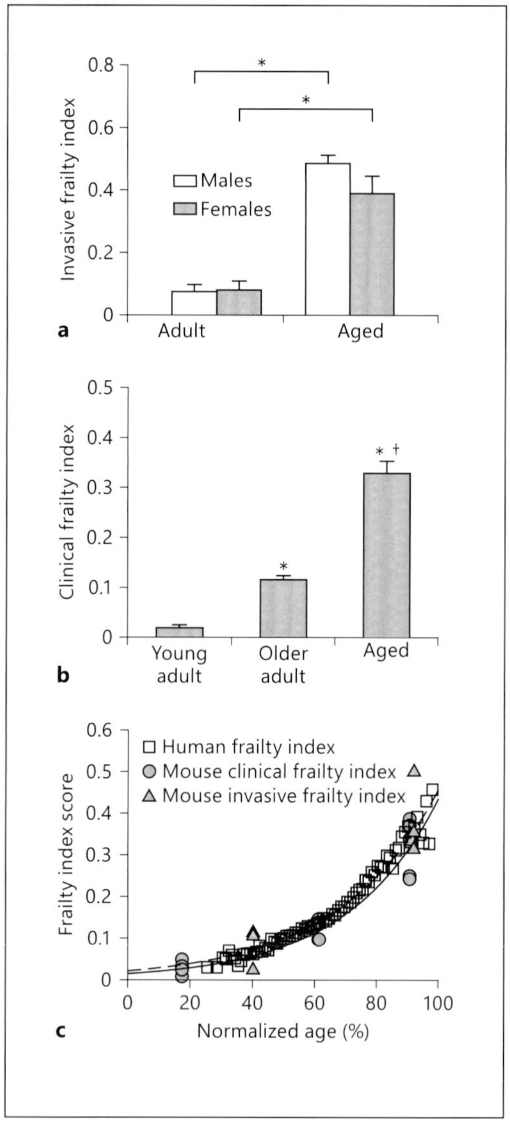

Fig. 1. Frailty index scores in mice of various ages compared with the frailty index data in humans. **a** The mean (±SEM) frailty index scores for 12-month-old (adult) and 30-month-old (aged) mice of both sexes illustrate the increase in frailty with age (n = 3 mice/group; * significantly different from the comparison group; $p < 0.001$). **b** The mean (±SEM) clinical frailty index scores increased with age [n = 5 young adult (~5-month-old), 4 older adult (~19-month-old) and 5 aged (~28-month-old) female mice; * significantly different from the young adults; † significantly different from the older adults; $p < 0.05$]. **c** The frailty index scores of humans from the Survey of Health, Ageing and Retirement in Europe (SHARE) survey were normalized to the age of 90% mortality of humans (open squares). The clinical frailty index scores (filled circles) and the invasive frailty index scores (filled triangles) of mice were normalized to the age of 90% mortality of mice. The frailty index increased exponentially with age in both humans ($r^2 = 0.97$; n = 30,025) and mice ($r^2 = 0.88$; n = 20). These data demonstrated that the relationship between the frailty index and age was similar between mice and humans. Panel A was reprinted from Parks et al. [25], and Panel B was reprinted from Whitehead et al. [26]. Panel C was modified from Whitehead et al. [26] using mouse invasive frailty index data from Parks et al. [25]. All figures are used with permission.

performance-based frailty index based on 8 noninvasive measures (e.g. activity levels and weight) could also be used to create a frailty index in mice. However, both the magnitude and the variance of the frailty index scores markedly increased when fewer items were measured, and this finding is similar to the results of studies in humans using a frailty index consisting of fewer than 30 variables [8]. Furthermore, this 8-item frailty index reflects only physical frailty.

To facilitate the use of the frailty index in both acute and longitudinal studies of aging mice, a procedure that is noninvasive, simple to implement, based on a broad range of parameters and based on a sufficient number of parameters (e.g. >30) is required to provide a robust estimate of frailty. Howlett et al. recently developed such a frailty index calculated from the clinical assessment of 31 potential deficits in aging mice [26]. These deficits were selected based on the assessment of established clinical signs of deterioration in mice [26]. Clinical assessment included evaluation of the integument, the musculoskeletal system, the ocular and nasal systems, the vestibulocochlear/auditory systems, the digestive system, the urogenital system, the respiratory system, signs of discomfort, body weight and body surface temperature. The severity of each deficit, except for body weight and temperature, was rated on a checklist with a simple 3-point scale. A score of 0 indicated no deficit, a score of 0.5 was given for a mild deficit, and a score of 1 was given for a severe deficit [26]. Deficits in body weight and body surface temperature were scored based on their deviation from reference values in young adult animals as described previously [25]. The values for each deficit were summed and divided by the total number of possible deficits to yield an individualized frailty index for each animal. The results of this study showed that the average murine frailty index scores significantly increased between the ages of 5 and 28 months (fig. 1b). These findings demonstrate that a simplified, noninvasive frailty index based on readily apparent signs of clinical deterioration can be used to quantify frailty in aging mice.

To validate the use of the clinical frailty index in translational studies, Whitehead et al. [26] directly compared features of the murine frailty index with those of the human frailty index. They used data from the Survey of Health, Ageing and Retirement in Europe (SHARE) database and calculated frailty index scores based on 70 self-reported measures in the survey, including data on physical health, behavioral risks, cognitive function and mental health [26]. To directly compare the relationship between the frailty index and age in mice and humans, age was normalized in each respective group to the age of 90% mortality for humans or mice. As shown in figure 1c, the frailty index increased exponentially with age in both humans and mice, and the relationship between the frailty index and normalized age was virtually identical between the two groups [26]. The work of Howlett et al. highlights other similarities between the clinical frailty index for mice and the frailty index for humans. The actual frailty index values for each age group in mice [25, 26] are similar to those in humans at comparable ages [2]. Furthermore, the rates of deficit accumulation, calculated from the slopes of the lines of the natural logarithm of the frailty index plotted as a function of age, were similar (~0.03) between mice and humans [26]. The highest frailty index score recorded in mice was close to 0.67, the submaximal limit of frailty reported in humans [8].

The work of Howlett et al. represents a new advance in the investigation of frailty in animal models. Their results show that a frailty index based on deficit accumulation can be developed for use in aging mice. Importantly, this index exhibits key features of the frailty index observed in clinical studies in humans. This frailty index based on deficit accumulation may be useful not only in studies of the biology of frailty in aging mice but also in other models of aging as well as in the assessment of frailty in genetically manipulated animals.

Summary

Frailty is a major problem in our aging society, as frail individuals have higher mortality and worse outcomes and use more health care services than age-matched individuals who are not frail. Thus, the need to explore the biology of frailty in preclinical models that mimic human frailty has been identified as a key step to promote translational research in this area. The newly developed models of frailty in animals described in this review are certain to accelerate basic research in the area of the biology of frailty. This recent progress in the identification and investigation of frailty in animal models is an important step forward in the effort to translate laboratory-based discoveries into clinical interventions.

References

1 Rockwood K, Fox RA, Stolee P, Robertson D, Beattie B: Frailty in elderly people: an evolving concept. CMAJ 1994;150:489–495.

2 Rockwood K, Song X, Mitnitski A: Changes in relative fitness and frailty across the adult lifespan: evidence from the Canadian National Population Health Survey. CMAJ 2012;183:E487–E494.

3 Rodríguez-Mañas L, Féart C, Mann G, Viña J, Chatterji S, Chodzko-Zajko W, Gonzalez-Colaço Harmand M, Bergman H, Carcaillon L, Nicholson C, Scuteri A, Sinclair A, Pelaez M, Van der Cammen T, Beland F, Bickenbach J, Delamarche P, Ferrucci L, Fried LP, Gutiérrez-Robledo LM, Rockwood K, Rodríguez Artalejo F, Serviddio G, Vega E; FOD-CC group (Appendix 1): Searching for an operational definition of frailty: a Delphi method based consensus statement: the frailty operative definition-consensus conference project. J Gerontol A Biol Sci Med Sci 2013;68:62–67.

4 Fulop T, Larbi A, Witkowski JM, McElhaney J, Loeb M, Mitnitski A, Pawelec G: Aging, frailty and age-related diseases. Biogerontology 2010;11:547–563.

5 de Vries NM, Staal JB, van Ravensberg CD, Hobbelen JS, Olde Rikkert MG, Nijhuis-van der Sanden MW: Outcome instruments to measure frailty: a systematic review. Ageing Res Rev 2011;10:104–114.

6 Fried LP, Tangen CM, Walston J, Newman AB, Hirsch C, Gottdiener J, Seeman T, Tracy R, Kop WJ, Burke G, McBurnie MA: Cardiovascular Health Study Collaborative Research Group: Frailty in older adults: evidence for a phenotype. J Gerontol A Biol Sci Med Sci 2001;56:M146–M156.

7 Mitnitski AB, Mogilner AJ, Rockwood K: Accumulation of deficits as a proxy measure of aging. Scientific World Journal 2001;1:323–336.

8 Clegg A, Young J, Iliffe S, Rikkert MO, Rockwood K: Frailty in elderly people. Lancet 2013;381:752–762.

9 Le Bourg E: Fasting can protect young and middle-aged Drosophila melanogaster flies against a severe cold stress. Biogerontology 2013;14:513–529.

10 McDonald P, Maizi BM, Arking R: Chemical regulation of mid- and late-life longevities in Drosophila. Exp Gerontol 2013;48:240–249.

11 Jones MA, Grotewiel M: Drosophila as a model for age-related impairment in locomotor and other behaviors. Exp Gerontol 2011;46:320–325.

12 Glenn CF, Chow DK, David L, Cooke CA, Gami MS, Iser WB, Hanselman KB, Goldberg IG, Wolkow CA: Behavioral deficits during early stages of aging in Caenorhabditis elegans result from locomotory deficits possibly linked to muscle frailty. J Gerontol A Biol Sci Med Sci 2004;59:1251–1260.

13 Mulcahy B, Holden-Dye L, O'Connor V: Pharmacological assays reveal age-related changes in synaptic transmission at the Caenorhabditis elegans neuromuscular junction that are modified by reduced insulin signalling. J Exp Biol 2013;216:492–501.

14 Iwasa H, Yu S, Xue J, Driscoll M: Novel EGF pathway regulators modulate C. elegans healthspan and lifespan via EGF receptor, PLC-gamma, and IP3R activation. Aging Cell 2010;9:490–505.

15 Ingram DK, Reynolds MA: Assessing the predictive validity of psychomotor tests as measures of biological age in mice. Exp Aging Res 1986;12:155–162.

16 Romanick M, Thompson LV, Brown-Borg HM: Murine models of atrophy, cachexia, and sarcopenia in skeletal muscle. Biochim Biophys Acta 2013;1832:1410–1420.

17 Weber H, Rauch A, Adamski S, Chakravarthy K, Kulkarni A, Dogdas B, Bendtsen C, Kath G, Alves SE, Wilkinson HA, Chiu CS: Automated rodent in situ muscle contraction assay and myofiber organization analysis in sarcopenia animal models. J Appl Physiol 2012;112:2087–2098.
18 Graber TG, Ferguson-Stegall L, Kim JH, Thompson LV: C57BL/6 neuromuscular healthspan scoring system. J Gerontol A Biol Sci Med Sci 2013;68:1326–1336.
19 Walston J, Hadley EC, Ferrucci L, Guralnik JM, Newman AB, Studenski SA, Ershler WB, Harris T, Fried LP: Research agenda for frailty in older adults: toward a better understanding of physiology and etiology: summary from the American Geriatrics Society/National Institute on Aging Research Conference on Frailty in Older Adults. J Am Geriatr Soc 2006;54:991–1001.
20 Walston J, Fedarko N, Yang H, Leng S, Beamer B, Espinoza S, Lipton A, Zheng H, Becker K: The physical and biological characterization of a frail mouse model. J Gerontol A Biol Sci Med Sci 2008;63:391–398.
21 Rennick DM, Fort MM: Lessons from genetically engineered animal models. XII. IL-10-deficient (IL-10(–/–) mice and intestinal inflammation. Am J Physiol Gastrointest Liver Physiol 2000;278:G829–G833.
22 Ko F, Yu Q, Xue QL, Yao W, Brayton C, Yang H, Fedarko N, Walston J: Inflammation and mortality in a frail mouse model. Age (Dordr) 2012;34:705–715.
23 Akki A, Yang H, Gupta A, Chacko VP, Yano T, Leppo MK, Steenbergen C, Walston J, Weiss RG: Skeletal muscle ATP kinetics are impaired in frail mice. Age (Dordr) 2014;36:21–30.
24 Sikka G, Miller KL, Steppan J, Pandey D, Jung SM, Fraser CD 3rd, Ellis C, Ross D, Vandegaer K, Bedja D, Gabrielson K, Walston JD, Berkowitz DE, Barouch LA: Interleukin 10 knockout frail mice develop cardiac and vascular dysfunction with increased age. Exp Gerontol 2013;48:128–135.
25 Parks RJ, Fares E, Macdonald JK, Ernst MC, Sinal CJ, Rockwood K, Howlett SE: A procedure for creating a frailty index based on deficit accumulation in aging mice. J Gerontol A Biol Sci Med Sci 2012;67:217–227.
26 Whitehead JC, Hildebrand BA, Sun M, Rockwood MR, Rose RA, Rockwood K, Howlett SE: A clinical frailty index in aging mice: comparisons with frailty index data in humans. J Gerontol A Biol Sci Med Sci 2014;69:621–632.

Susan E. Howlett, PhD
Department of Pharmacology, Dalhousie University
Sir Charles Tupper Medical Building, 5850 College Street
PO Box 15000, Halifax, NS B3H 4R2 (Canada)
E-Mail Susan.Howlett@dal.ca

Theou O, Rockwood K (eds): Frailty in Aging. Biological, Clinical and Social Implications.
Interdiscipl Top Gerontol Geriatr. Basel, Karger, 2015, vol 41, pp 26–40 (DOI: 10.1159/000381134)

Frailty, Inflammation and Immunosenescence

Tamas Fulop[a, c] • Janet McElhaney[d] • Graham Pawelec[h] • Alan A. Cohen[b, c] • José A. Morais[f, g] • Gilles Dupuis[a, c] • Sarra Baehl[a, c] • Xavier Camous[i] • Jacek M. Witkowski[j] • Anis Larbi[i]

[a]Geriatrics Division, Department of Medicine and [b]Department of Family Medicine and [c]Research Center on Aging, Faculty of Medicine and Health Sciences, University of Sherbrooke, Sherbrooke, Que., and [d]Advanced Medical Research Institute of Canada, Sudbury, Ont., and [e]Division of Geriatric Medicine, Department of Medicine and [f]McGill Nutrition and Food Science Centre and [g]Royal Victoria Hospital, McGill University Health Centre, McGill University, Montreal, Que., Canada; [h]Center for Medical Research, University of Tübingen, Tübingen, Germany; [i]Singapore Immunology Network (SIgN), Biopolis, Agency for Science Technology and Research (A*STAR), Singapore, Singapore; [j]Department of Pathophysiology, Medical University of Gdansk, Gdansk, Poland

Abstract

Frailty is a still-evolving concept of a complex phenomenon. There are several algorithms and strategies for assessing frailty syndrome, but currently, no universally accepted definition or measurement protocol has been determined. Consequently, the biological cause(s) of frailty are also poorly defined. Much circumstantial experimental data point to the dysregulation of several key physiological systems, including the neuroendocrine, musculoskeletal, metabolic and immune/inflammatory systems, resulting from alterations in functional reserves. Immune dysregulation and inflammation as causes of frailty have gained some support from the results of longitudinal studies, but a true causal relationship has not been established. This chapter will describe the immune/inflammatory alterations found in frailty and their putative causal relationships with this state.

Over the last decade, one of the most important conceptual advances in geriatrics has been the establishment of the concept of frailty [1–5]. Its identification has stimulated a huge body of research to identify its causes and to better define it clinically. The prevalence of frailty, as determined by the Cardiovascular Health Study (CHS) in a population aged >65 years, is estimated to be about 7%, and it characteristically increases with age [1]. Similar data have been reported by other large longitudinal studies [6]. There are currently many ways to approach frailty conceptually and to define it clinically [7–9]. Several key physiological systems are involved in the frailty trajectory, including the musculoskeletal, hormonal, metabolic and immune-inflammatory systems, with the additional cautious inclusion of cognitive parameters [1, 10–12]. There is at least some experimental evidence that an immune component of frailty exists [13, 14]. The relationships between the phenotype of frailty and commonly measured molecular and cellular inflammatory markers are increasingly being documented [15, 16]. However, the real question is whether these measured markers play determinant causal roles in the pathogenesis of frailty or whether they are caused by this state. Here, we will discuss how frailty can be defined biologically and what the contribution of the immune-inflammatory system could be.

How Can We Define Aging and Frailty?

There is currently no universally accepted definition for either aging or frailty. The definitions differ depending on the dimension in which they are conceptualized, for example, at the population, individual, research or clinical level.

The Aging Process

To define and understand aging, we have considered more than 200 existing theories that are mainly speculative, with little or no supporting experimental evidence. Taken together, these theories suggest that we have only a partial understanding of the aging phenomenon. It is now quite clear that aging can be defined in many ways, such as from a genetic perspective or from a stochastic perspective [17]. Some characteristics of the aging process seem to be widely accepted, such as its universality, dependence on time, irreversibility, and culmination in death. Nevertheless, inter-individual differences in longevity and disease susceptibility suggest that certain components can be modulated to delay the onset of frailty toward the end of life without really impacting the final outcome (i.e. mortality) [18].

Another definition, which is more physiological and perhaps more relevant to humans and can be operationalized in the clinic, involves various systems and their functionalities (fig. 1). In this context, we can define aging as continuous changes (mainly erosions) in several physiological systems in parallel, either independently from one another or not and converging toward the exhaustion of intrinsic reserves, rendering the organism more susceptible to all kinds and severities of stress (fig. 2). Thus, elderly individuals become more susceptible to the effects of stress compared to young subjects, who are able to cope efficiently with the same type and intensity of stress. It is worth mentioning that the intensity and repetition of the stress is very important, as suggested by the theory of hormesis, which states that multiple, low-intensity stimulations lead to adaptation compared to a unique high-intensity stimulation, which may have serious impacts and even result in death. Taking this theory into consideration, the consequence for humans is that after each of these episodes, recovery may be slower, and most of the time, it is only partial. This definition heavily relies on the existence of physiologic reserves because recovery ultimately depends on the level of remaining reserves. The greater the

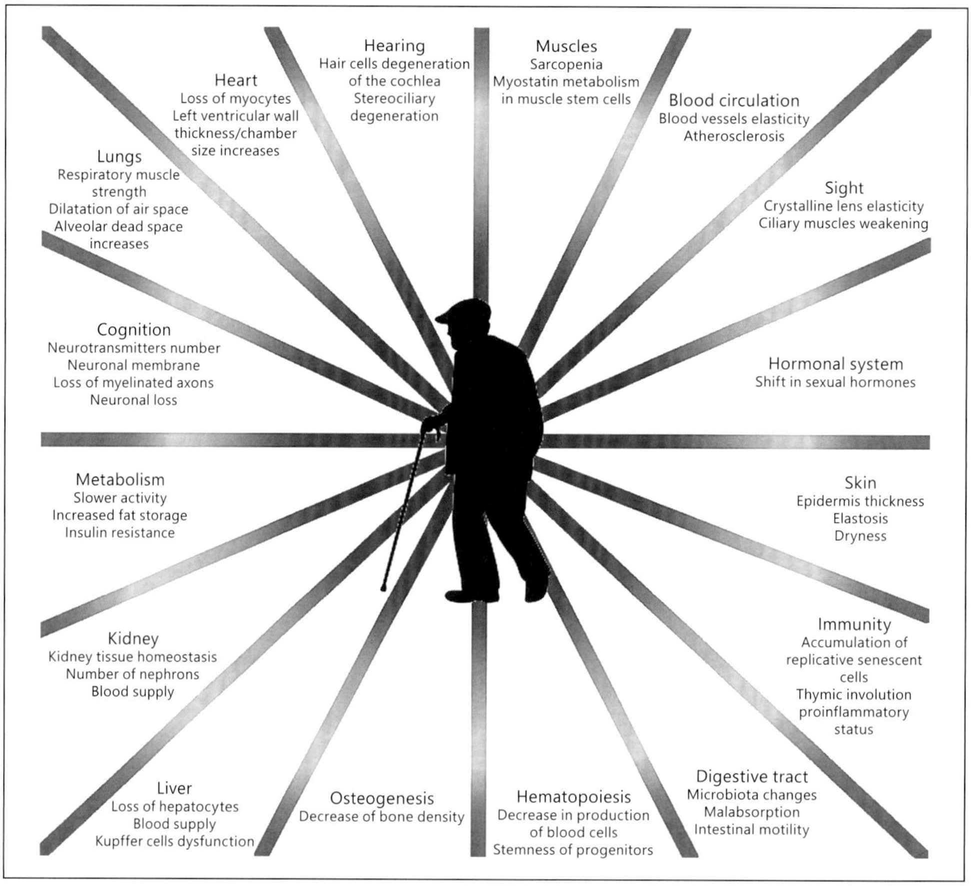

Fig. 1. Dysfunctionality occurring during aging, assuming the absence of both co-morbidities and the adverse effects of medications.

level of biological reserves, the better recovery will be. It has to be noted that the biological reserves that we are referring to are a compilation of the different functional systems of an organism, especially those showing age-related erosion. This information directly implies that if the original reserve is low, as occurs with the aging process, even a minor challenge to this already eroded system will result in functional failure, allowing the initiation of various syndromes and leading to the development of physical dependence. Concomitant with this loss of physiological reserves due to the aging process *per se*, susceptibility to the development of other co-morbidities increases (chronic diseases, such as dementia, cancer, and cardio-vascular diseases). As such, these chronic diseases are either the consequences or simply the clinical manifestations of the loss of reserves due to aging. Although many scientists consider aging to be a disease, accumulating evidence concerning aging suggests that it is not a disease, it is a physiological process that increases susceptibility to disease. In this same conceptual framework, the notion of frailty has been introduced to distinguish physiological aging from chronic diseases [19].

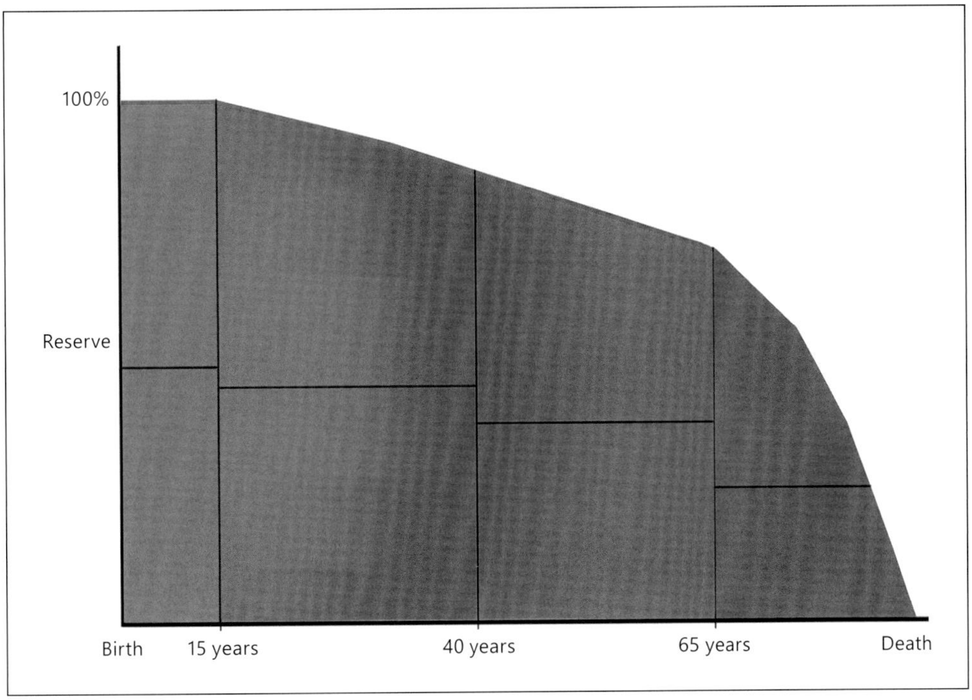

Fig. 2. Model of biological aging. Model of aging, showing the progressive biological and immunological changes that occur with time and their impacts on the body's reserves. In this model, the reserves are considered empty at the moment of death.

Frailty as a Syndrome or State

The current consensus on the definition and understanding of frailty is that because of its multicausal nature, it is a complex phenomenon resulting from the cumulative erosion of reserves in multiple physiological systems and organs manifested by homeostenosis [1, 2]. This physiologic dysregulation is observed on a complex systems level, involving several organ systems, including the musculoskeletal, immune, endocrine, hematologic, and cardiovascular systems [3, 10, 20]. This multi-organ dysregulation (fig. 1) is triggered or revealed by minor stressor events or stimuli, and its complexity may also lie in the variety of stressors that may be responsible for its initiation and progression. The consequences of this multi-organ 'failure' are more important than the dysregulation displayed at the level of each individual system [19]. Ultimately, it may result in greater vulnerability to some serious adverse outcomes, such as falls, institutionalization and death. Finally, and most importantly, age plays a major role in this dysregulation, consequently resulting in an increased disease prevalence with age. Currently accumulated data strongly suggest that 'true' frailty is an extension of the physiological aging process, being at the cross-roads of biological age and the manifestation of chronic age-related diseases [19]. In this way, as already suggested, frailty is the reflection and manifestation of the biological age of a subject, which can evolve in many directions depending on the nature of the stresses experienced [19].

There are several operational approaches for defining frailty, particularly as a syndrome applicable at the clinical level and not only as a theoretical concept. One of the most commonly used definitions is that developed by Fried et al. [1], whose phenotypic description of frailty is based on the presence or absence of very specific physical components related to physical fitness and metabolism. According to this definition, the major criteria for characterizing the phenotype of frailty as a clinical syndrome are the following: unintentional weight loss, weakness, exhaustion, slowed walking speed and a low physical activity level. An individual with three or more of these characteristics is considered frail, while the presence of one or two of them indicates a pre-frailty state, and the absence of all five indicates a nonfrail state. The other most often used definition of frailty is a much more holistic and multidimensional approach that was first described by Rockwood et al. [2, 20]. In their conceptualized definition, frailty is viewed as a state of the accumulation of functional deficits, extending well beyond the physical definition of Fried and potentially including cognitive decline, chronic diseases, environmental risk factors, psycho-social risk factors, geriatric syndromes (e.g. falls, delirium, and urinary incontinence) and even age-related disabilities. These two definitions of frailty, despite consisting of different components, some of which have been highly debated (e.g. cognitive decline), are largely complementary for use by clinical professionals.

How can we practically measure frailty? Obviously, its measurement differs according to the type of conceptualization of frailty syndrome applied. According to Fried et al.'s definition, frailty is measured using a clinical score ranging from 0 to 5, while for that of Rockwood et al., it is measured by accumulating as many components as possible (currently including around 30–40 parameters). However, other methods are also in use, such as the Clinical Frailty Scale, which is more easily applied in the clinical setting but is much less sensitive to change in frailty compared to corresponding changes in the frailty index [21]. Currently, each method has some advantages and disadvantages relative to the others, and their uses depend on the clinical and/or research setting in which they are applied.

Another way to conceptualize frailty has recently emerged, in which it is considered as 'primary' or 'secondary' [19, 22]. Primary frailty signifies that it is not associated with any specific disease or functional decline causing incapacity. In this context, this type of frailty is considered an extension of the physiological aging process in which an older person is even more susceptible to an adverse outcome than what normal aging would predict. On the other hand, frailty may be defined as secondary when it is clearly associated with underlying diseases that are for the most part chronic or related to physical incapacity. Taken together, these various approaches to frailty suggest that there is not one syndrome but different levels and forms of frailty resulting from the convergence of different numbers of pathways, all of which are more or less influenced by aging.

What Is the Cause of Frailty?

Having defined frailty as a cumulative decline and loss of physiological reserves in multiple organs and systems, the question arises as to whether any system is more important than the others to the development of frailty or whether each contributes equally. Studies conducted in the last few years have suggested that the immune/inflammatory system may play a more important role in frailty development than any other system [13–15]. This finding may sound counter-intuitive because most of the eroded components' functions in frailty are linked to physical/metabolic pathways. We will describe how immune/inflammatory alterations may contribute to frailty in the following sections.

Immunosenescence and Inflamm-Aging

Aging is associated with changes in the immune system that are collectively designated as 'immunosenescence' [23]. The immune system fundamentally determines how an organism is able to combat different extrinsic and intrinsic challenges. Elderly people are more susceptible to infections, cancers and autoimmune disorders. The cause of this susceptibility is likely to at least partly involve alterations in both the innate and adaptive immune systems that have been observed in all mammals studied to date [24].

The innate immune system, which is composed of different cell types, such as neutrophils, monocytes/macrophages, dendritic cells and natural killer cells, is altered with aging. The most important function of the innate immune system is to be the first line of protection for an organism against various invaders. Most of the time, this line of defense is enough to eradicate the danger. Because microorganisms are usually phylogenetically conserved, their pathogen-associated molecular patterns are highly conserved and are not shared by mammals; thus, they can be recognized as nonself by nonpolymorphic activating receptors expressed on the surfaces of innate immune cells. Innate immune responses strongly influence subsequent adaptive immune responses via antigen processing and presentation and cytokine and chemokine production. It is now well accepted that the effector functions of cells of the innate immune response are decreased with aging. Phagocytosis, chemotaxis, free radical production and antigen presentation are all altered, but to different extents. Therefore, the first line of defense against aggressors is compromised with aging. It should be mentioned that as a consequence of continuous antigenic stimulation, these cells evolve in a pro-inflammatory environment that exists in the quiescent state of aged individuals. This constant stimulation is accompanied by increases in the production of free radicals and pro-inflammatory cytokines, including TNF and IL-6, which may cause 'collateral damage' to host tissues. This basal activation results in the deregulation of other physiological systems, such as the musculoskeletal, cardiovascular and neuroendocrine systems [25]. These immune functions are mediated by the activation of cells following ligation of their membrane receptors, but the numbers of most of these receptors are not changed with aging. Thus, changes in signaling pathways have been discovered, explaining the functional alterations in the presence of unchanged receptor numbers. Many signaling pathways, such as the Jak/STAT, PI3K and MAPK pathways, are altered under stimulatory conditions with aging and also explain the altered susceptibility to apoptosis.

Studies of gene regulation in monocytes in relation to frailty have shown the upregulation of the *ex vivo* expression of seven stress-responsive inflammatory pathway genes upon lipopolysaccharide stimulation, including transcription factors, signal transduction proteins, chemokines (CXCL10) and cytokines, which are concomitantly upregulated with stress-sensitive genes. Thus, changes in the innate immune response with aging lead to increased incidences of infections, cancers and autoimmune disorders due to a basal state of inflammatory activation and the lack of an adequate immune response under stimulation [24]. One of the notable consequences of these changes is the alteration of the adaptive immune response.

The adaptive immune response is currently considered to be the most severely affected immune response by aging, as reflected by changes in the phenotypes and functions of both B and T cells [23]. Due to chronic antigenic stimulation, T cells undergo a process of differentiation/exhaustion, leading to the accumulation of memory cells specific for previously encountered antigens. The best example of this process is persistent cytomegalovirus (CMV) infection, which drives the accumulation of late-differentiated CD8+ T cells specific for CMV (fig. 3) [26]. These CMV-specific CD8+ T cells help to prevent CMV reactivation by killing virus-infected cells, thereby controlling virus replication at the expense of immune exhaustion. Nonetheless, a Swedish longitudinal study has shown that the accumulation of these CMV-specific CD8+ T cells is part of a cluster of risk factors that has been shown to be correlated with mortality at 2-, 4- and 6-year follow-ups of the very elderly, and these results have led to the definition of the immune risk profile [27]. These findings further reinforce the role of the adaptive immune system in the determination of the longevity of elderly people. Not only do these memory cells accumulate with aging and fill the 'immune space', their specific functions, including clonal expansion, IL-2 production and their abilities to help T cells with specific effector functions, are altered. These functional changes are related to alterations in signaling pathways, including T cell receptor, CD28 and cytokine receptor signaling. Furthermore, suppressive regulatory T cells, seem to be more active in the elderly than in young individuals. These alterations, together with the changes in the innate immune response, create a state of low-grade inflammation dubbed 'inflamm-aging' [28]. This state is fertile soil for the development of chronic inflammatory diseases in relation to the aging process.

Interestingly, some studies have focused on neopterin determination as a surrogate of viral infection. It has been well established that some aspects of immunosenescence may be attributed to the increased latent CMV infection prevalence with aging [23]. This increase considerably affects the phenotypic distribution of the CD8 compartment. A study of community-dwelling older adults has found that elevated neopterin

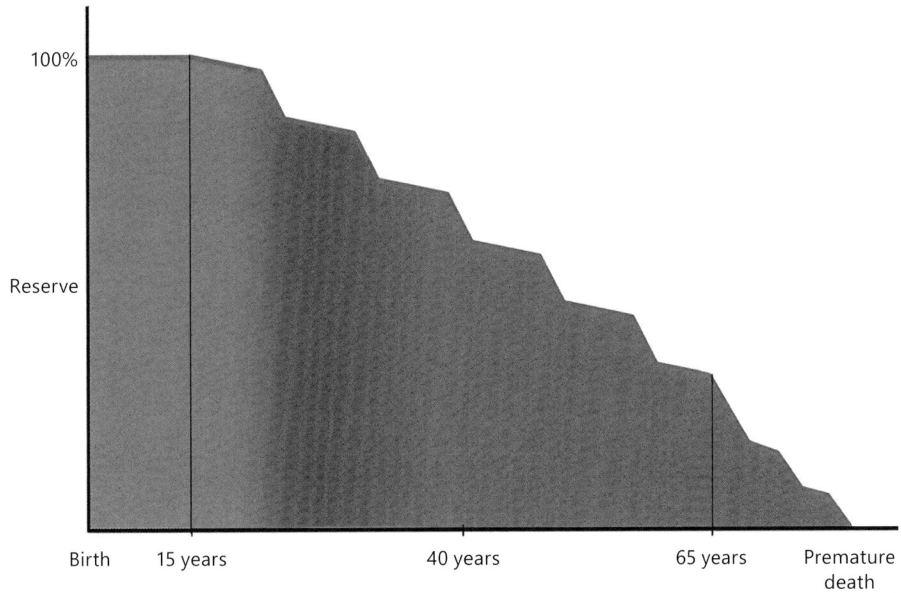

Fig. 3. Impact of continuous antigenic/immune stimulation on the aging process: a model of accelerated biological aging. Constant immune surveillance against persistent infections is essential for survival despite the heavy costs, resulting in decreased biological reserves. This process leads to a state of insufficient reserves preceding death. This period of time may be called frailty.

levels and CMV are associated with frailty, independent of IL-6 levels [29]; however, this finding could not be confirmed in other studies [30].

In addition, direct alterations occur in the adaptive immune system in relation to frailty that are considered to be part of the immune/inflammatory process. Frail women have significantly higher CD8+ and CD8+CD28- T cell counts than nonfrail elderly women. In another study, frail individuals have been demonstrated to have an increased T cell subpopulation expressing the CCR5 receptor, which contributes to the pro-inflammatory condition in frailty. A decreased CD4:CD8 ratio has also been identified in these individuals [13]. These alterations in cellular immunity further contribute to the inflammatory status that is initiated and sustained by the innate immune system in frailty.

Together, the bulk of the studies that have been conducted to elucidate the putative causes of frailty have suggested that significant monocyte/macrophage-mediated immune activation marked by elevated cell numbers, genetic markers, IL-6 production and neopterin levels occurs in frail older adults. As previously mentioned, the T cell compartment is also heavily influenced by latent CMV infection, which leads to increases in specific memory T cells and TEMRA clones. However, there is no clear conceptualization of how these T cell changes further contribute to the sustained

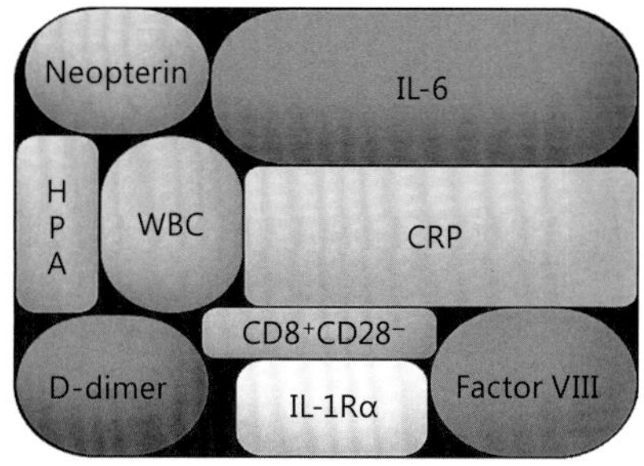

Fig. 4. Immune/inflammatory components of frailty.

inflammation induced by the innate immune system. These data highlight the putative role of the innate immune response in promoting low-grade inflammation in association with aging, which eventually becomes even more dysregulated, resulting in frailty (fig. 4). Furthermore, these inflammatory alterations that occur through various pathways may induce the appearance of chronic diseases, increased disability and even increased mortality.

Our preliminary data from a large longitudinal study conducted in Singapore only partially confirmed these findings, in which the frequencies of some memory CD8+ T cells have been found to be associated with frailty (unpublished data). When the frailty score based on Fried et al.'s definition was broken down into individual components, these changes disappeared compared to the use of the 5-component score. Other studies have also recently found conflicting results compared to those of the above-mentioned studies, namely with regard to neopterin, white blood cells (WBCs) and IL-6. These results bring into question the predominant role of immune/inflammatory pathways in the development of frailty. In line with the results of our study, the Newcastle 85+ study could not demonstrate an association of CMV sero-positivity, telomere length, markers of oxidative stress or DNA damage or repair with frailty or an inverse association of frailty with the memory/naïve CD8+ T cell ratio.

Taken together, the changes in the adaptive immune response with aging further contribute to the higher incidences of infections, cancers and autoimmune disorders in addition to the development of chronic inflammatory diseases, such as neurodegenerative and cardiovascular diseases. The question is whether these immune changes associated with aging may contribute to the development of frailty.

Immune Frailty

With aging, alterations in the immune system and the emergence of frailty occur. Several studies (mainly longitudinal) have suggested that one of the most important pathways in the development of frailty is the immune/inflammatory pathway (fig. 4) [1–15].

Longitudinal studies, such as the InCHIANTI study, have found that high levels of IL-6, IL-1ra and C-reactive protein (CRP) are significantly associated with poor overall physical performance, reduced muscle strength and central obesity [31]. The EPESE study has demonstrated age-associated increases in IL-6, D-dimer, factor VIII and fibrinogen and has shown that IL-6 and D-dimer are predictive of mortality. The Longitudinal Aging Study of Amsterdam (LASA) has identified a high level of CRP as a risk factor for frailty. The Women's Health and Aging Study has found that the WBC count and IL-6 level are higher in frail vs. nonfrail individuals. Finally, the Health ABC study has found that elevated levels of IL-6 and TNF are inversely associated with muscle mass and strength. The Newcastle 85+ study has confirmed the importance of these inflammatory markers in frailty [32].

The alterations described in the innate and adaptive immune systems lead to the disequilibrium of the immune response, resulting in low-grade inflammation associated with the aging process [28]. From the aforementioned studies, the notion has emerged that immune and inflammatory alterations are causative of frailty development [13–15]. The inflammatory process of frailty is characterized by increases in the levels of pro-inflammatory cytokines, such as IL-6, as well as the CRP level and WBC count. Further, the age-related activation of the coagulation system and increases in the levels of pro-coagulant markers along with the activities of atherosclerotic processes associated with aging implicate D-dimers, factor VIII, fibrinogen and plasminogen-activating inhibitor-1 in this inflammatory process [15]. Correspondingly, these markers have also been found to be associated with the development of frailty in connection with inflammatory markers [13–15], as has been shown by the CHS. Immune/inflammatory changes can also directly or indirectly lead to many other deleterious consequences through alterations in other physiological systems, either sequentially or in parallel. These alterations may affect the neuroendocrine system, resulting in the decreased production of hormones, such as IGF-1, the metabolic system, resulting in altered protein and lipid metabolism and finally, the hematopoietic system, resulting in decreased hemoglobin levels, all contributing to manifestations of frailty.

One central node of these alterations could be an increase in the level of the pro-inflammatory cytokine IL-6. IL-6 is known to have pleiotropic effects and has been independently associated with frailty [33]. It substantially contributes to various characteristics observed in frail older individuals, such as anemia, decreased lean body mass or sarcopenia, osteoporosis, the hypothalamo-hypophyseal-adrenal axis, manifested as increased cortisol and adrenaline production, and alterations in the humoral and cellular immune responses. IL-6 has been shown to independently predict steeper functional decline during a follow-up of 3.5 years [34], as measured by decreased muscle strength and power and slowed walking speed, which are two central components of frailty syndrome. Furthermore, IL-6 has been associated with atherosclerosis, osteoporosis and sarcopenia, leading to functional decline, the development of disabilities and all-cause mortality. An *in vitro* study has shown that peripheral blood mononuclear cells stimulated by lipopolysaccharides produce more IL-6 in frail compared to nonfrail community-dwelling subjects. Thus, IL-6 may have a central role in the development of frailty. In contrast, the LASA has failed to demonstrate any relationship between serum IL-6 levels and either baseline or incident frailty. In any case, one must bear in mind that because frailty remains an ill-defined clinical concept, there is no study demonstrating a causative effect of IL-6 on its occurrence.

As alluded to above, one other common inflammatory marker associated with or being considered in frailty is CRP, which has been shown by the CHS and the LASA to be a cardiovascular disease risk factor independently associated with frailty. Further, the combination of CRP with IL-6 seems to have a greater effect. IL-6 and CRP alone and in combination have been associated with mortality in healthy older adults, as demonstrated by an IL-6 level of >3.19 pg/μl, yielding a risk ratio (RR) of 2.1 (CI 1.3–3.4), a CRP level of >2.78 mg/l, with an RR of 1.7, (CI 1.1–2.6), and both markers together yielding an RR of 3.5 (CI 1.4–5.4) [13–15].

Although sarcopenia has not been directly associated with the frailty phenotype, it is an indirectly essential component [35]. The exact cause of sarcopenia is not known; however, mediators of inflammation seem to largely contribute to its pathogenesis. Notably, direct experimental evidence incriminating inflammation in the development of sarcopenia is lacking in humans. Most of our knowledge again comes from various epidemiological data. The InCHIANTI study has found that high levels of IL-6, IL1ra and CRP are significantly associated with poor overall physical performance and reduced muscle strength, indicating reduced muscle mass (sarcopenia) [34]. The same results have been obtained in the Framingham Heart Study and in the Health ABC study. In addition, decreasing muscle mass causes an increase in fat mass, further contributing to the inflammatory status (via adipokines) and resulting in functional decline and disability.

The next parameter associated with frailty is the WBC count [33]. An elevated WBC count that is within the normal range is associated with cardiovascular and cerebrovascular events, cardiovascular and cancer mortality, and all-cause mortality in older adults. Direct relationships of frailty with elevated WBC, neutrophil and monocyte counts have been reported. The prevalence of Fried frailty was found to be increased at the 2003–2005 follow-ups according to the biomarker distribution observed at the 1994–1995 baseline in the Hertfordshire Aging Study [11]. In the CHS, nonfrail participants were assessed at baseline and then after 5 and 9 years for the development of frailty, and the total WBC counts concomitant with the CRP and IL-6 levels were each found to be associated with an increased risk of frailty. However, after adjusting for confounders, only the CRP remained significant. The Women's Health and Aging Study I has revealed that the odds of being frail vs. nonfrail or prefrail, as determined by comparing the top and middle tertiles for neutrophil or monocyte cell counts and IL-6 levels, are increased (n = 558) [33]. It should be mentioned that these findings were obtained by assessing community-dwelling older adults with a high prevalence of functional disability, which may have masked several underlying undiagnosed chronic diseases. The findings of these studies suggest that neutrophils and monocytes have potential roles in the pathogenesis of frailty, most probably via the generation and maintenance of an inflammatory status.

Other immune-neuroendocrine-inflammatory parameters have also been associated with frailty. Among the coagulation parameters, factor VIII, tissue plasminogen activators and fibrin D-dimer have been related to frailty in several studies [15]. Considering the oxidative stress parameters, increases in serum 8-hydroxydesoxyguanosin, oxidized glutathione, malonaldehyde and 4-hydroxynonenal and protein adducts and a decline in the powerful antioxidant thioredoxin have been associated with frailty [36]. Levels of the immune-associated hormones ghrelin, IGF-1 and vitamin D have also been shown to be decreased during the development of frailty, corresponding with increases in inflammatory markers and the altered homeostases of hormones, including IGF-1, testosterone, and thyroid hormones [35]. The hemoglobin and glucose levels are additional parameters that should be considered in relation to the immune/inflammatory process [37]. More recently identified surrogates of inflamm-aging and frailty include total circulating cell-free DNA and its unmethylated content, while the plasma mitochondrial DNA concentration has been found to be a marker of the physical aspect of frailty in a study of nonagenarians [38]. However, there is very little information on the roles of these markers in the development of frailty.

How Can We Conceptualize Immune/Inflammation in the Pathogenesis of Frailty? Unique or Integrative Approach

Frailty is a complex clinical concept, and it may be difficult to believe that it can be completely explained by one group of pathways, such as the immune/inflammatory pathways, despite the interconnectedness of these pathways with other systems. If the genesis of other geriatric syndromes is considered to be largely multifactorial, the case of frailty should be similar.

Frailty is largely an outcome of the activities of the pathways of many interacting and somehow dysregulated physiological systems. The functioning of these systems is determined by the effects of physiological aging and genetic background and mainly by environmental factors, including physical activity, high levels, nutritional factors and substance abuse. The interactions of these triggers with the unfavorable background created by the aging process results in the dysregulation of several systems, including the immune/inflammatory, neuroendocrine, cardiovascular, respiratory, renal, musculoskeletal and metabolic systems. This dysregulation manifests itself either spontaneously or under minimal stress as a frailty syndrome, such as anorexia, anemia, sarcopenia, osteoporosis, hyperglycemia or increased clotting, which can be assessed by the various frailty measures. Thus, the immune/inflammatory process is largely manifested as a catabolic metabolic cascade, from which the syndrome of frailty evolves. Frailty further results in exceptionally increased susceptibility to falls, delirium, institutionalization and even death.

Conclusions

Frailty syndrome, if we accept that it exists, seems to represent an intermediate state between the usual aging process and its impact on the progression of chronic diseases. Thus, frailty may represent the expression of a threshold in older people at which the exhaustion of the physiological reserve is at a critically advanced stage. Furthermore, it is more the result of the additive effects of altered systems than of abnormalities in one particular system, such as the immune/inflammatory, neuroendocrine, musculoskeletal or cardiovascular system. Frailty can be considered the expression of biological age rather than chronological age. However, the causal relationships between IL-6, TNF and other inflammatory markers and frailty have yet to be proven. Nevertheless, the immune/inflammatory hypothesis is very appealing and currently provides a biological framework for frailty, in an attempt to cover all aspects of the clinical frailty phenotype. More studies aiming to reveal the direct involvement of immune/inflammatory alterations in the pathogenesis of frailty are needed, with or without the re-definition of frailty syndrome. If we want to intervene either to prevent frailty or to slow its onset, we need to better understand the aging process and how the physiological reserves of an organism can be improved – keeping the glass half full!

Acknowledgments

This work was partly supported by grants from the Canadian Institutes of Health Research (CIHR) (No. 106634 and No. 106701), the Université de Sherbrooke, and the Research Center on Aging. X. Camous and A. Larbi are funded by the Singapore Immunology Network (SIgN) and the Agency for Science Technology and Research (A*STAR). A. Larbi is an ISAC Scholar.

References

1 Fried LP, Tangen CM, Walston J, Newman AB, Hirsch C, Gottdiener J, Seeman T, Tracy R, Kop WJ, Burke G, McBurnie MA; Cardiovascular Health Study Collaborative Research Group: Frailty in older adults: evidence for a phenotype. J Gerontol A Biol Sci Med Sci 2001;56:M146–M156.
2 Rockwood K, Andrew M, Mitnitski A: A comparison of two approaches to measuring frailty in elderly people. J Gerontol A Biol Sci Med Sci 2007;62:738–743.
3 Lacas A, Rockwood K: Frailty in primary care: a review of its conceptualization and implications for practice. BMC Med 2012;10:4.
4 Sternberg SA, Wershof Schwartz A, Karunananthan S, Bergman H, Mark Clarfield A: The identification of frailty: a systematic literature review. J Am Geriatr Soc 2011;59:2129–2138.
5 Rodríguez-Mañas L, Féart C, Mann G, Viña J, Chatterji S, Chodzko-Zajko W, Gonzalez-Colaço Harmand M, Bergman H, Carcaillon L, Nicholson C, Scuteri A, Sinclair A, Pelaez M, Van der Cammen T, Beland F, Bickenbach J, Delamarche P, Ferrucci L, Fried LP, Gutiérrez-Robledo LM, Rockwood K, Rodríguez Artalejo F, Serviddio G, Vega E; FOD-CC group (Appendix 1): Searching for an operational definition of frailty: a Delphi method based consensus statement: the frailty operative definition-consensus conference project. J Gerontol A Biol Sci Med Sci 2013;68:62–67.
6 Collard RM, Boter H, Schoevers RA, Oude Voshaar RC: Prevalence of frailty in community-dwelling older persons: a systematic review. J Am Geriatr Soc 2012;60:1487–1492.

7 Pijpers E, Ferreira I, Stehouwer CD, Nieuwenhuijzen Kruseman AC: The frailty dilemma. Review of the predictive accuracy of major frailty scores. Eur J Intern Med 2012;23:118–123.
8 Woo J, Leung J, Morley JE: Comparison of frailty indicators based on clinical phenotype and the multiple deficit approach in predicting mortality and physical limitation. J Am Geriatr Soc 2012;60:1478–1486.
9 Sourial N, Bergman H, Karunananthan S, Wolfson C, Payette H, Gutierrez-Robledo LM, Béland F, Fletcher JD, Guralnik J: Implementing frailty into clinical practice: a cautionary tale. J Gerontol A Biol Sci Med Sci 2013;68:1505–1511.
10 Ho YY, Matteini AM, Beamer B, Fried L, Xue QL, Arking DE, Chakravarti A, Fallin MD, Walston J: Exploring biologically relevant pathways in frailty. J Gerontol A Biol Sci Med Sci 2011;66:975–979.
11 Baylis D, Bartlett DB, Syddall HE, Ntani G, Gale CR, Cooper C, Lord JM, Sayer AA: Immune-endocrine biomarkers as predictors of frailty and mortality: a 10-year longitudinal study in community-dwelling older people. Age (Dordr) 2013;35:963–971.
12 Sandri M, Barberi L, Bijlsma AY, Blaauw B, Dyar KA, Milan G, Mammucari C, Meskers CG, Pallafacchina G, Paoli A, Pion D, Roceri M, Romanello V, Serrano AL, Toniolo L, Larsson L, Maier AB, Muñoz-Cánoves P, Musarò A, Pende M, Reggiani C, Rizzuto R, Schiaffino S: Signalling pathways regulating muscle mass in ageing skeletal muscle: the role of the IGF1-Akt-mTOR-FoxO pathway. Biogerontology 2013;14:303–323.
13 Yao X, Li H, Leng SX: Inflammation and immune system alterations in frailty. Clin Geriatr Med 2011; 27:79–87.
14 Chang SS, Weiss CO, Xue QL, Fried LP: Association between inflammatory-related disease burden and frailty: results from the Women's Health and Aging Studies (WHAS) I and II. Arch Gerontol Geriatr 2012;54:9–15.
15 Kanapuru B, Ershler WB: Inflammation, coagulation, and the pathway to frailty. Am J Med 2009;122: 605–613.
16 Fedarko NS: The biology of aging and frailty. Clin Geriatr Med 2011;27:27–37.
17 Kirkwood TB, Melov S: On the programmed/non-programmed nature of ageing within the life history. Curr Biol 2011;21:R701–R707.
18 Strehler BL, Mildvan AS: General theory of mortality and aging. Science 1960;132:14–21.
19 Fulop T, Larbi A, Witkowski JM, McElhaney J, Loeb M, Mitnitski A, Pawelec G: Aging, frailty and age-related diseases. Biogerontology 2010;11:547–563.
20 Rockwood K, Mitnitski A: Frailty defined by deficit accumulation and geriatric medicine defined by frailty. Clin Geriatr Med 2011;27:17–26.
21 Mitnitski A, Fallah N, Rockwood MR, Rockwood K: Transitions in cognitive status in relation to frailty in older adults: a comparison of three frailty measures. J Nutr Health Aging 2011;15:863–867.
22 Strandberg TE, Pitkälä KH: Frailty in elderly people. Lancet 2007;369:1328–1329.
23 Fülöp T, Larbi A, Pawelec G: Human T cell aging and the impact of persistent viral infections. Front Immunol 2013;4:271.
24 Fulop T, Fortin C, Lesur O, Dupuis G, Kotb R, Lord JM, Larbi A: The innate immune system and aging: what is the contribution to immunosenescence? Open Longevity Sci 2012;6:121–132.
25 Candore G, Caruso C, Jirillo E, Magrone T, Vasto S: Low grade inflammation as a common pathogenetic denominator in age-related diseases: novel drug targets for anti-ageing strategies and successful ageing achievement. Curr Pharm Des 2010;16:584–596.
26 Solana R, Tarazona R, Aiello AE, Akbar AN, Appay V, Beswick M, Bosch JA, Campos C, Cantisán S, Cicin-Sain L, Derhovanessian E, Ferrando-Martínez S, Frasca D, Fulöp T, Govind S, Grubeck-Loebenstein B, Hill A, Hurme M, Kern F, Larbi A, López-Botet M, Maier AB, McElhaney JE, Moss P, Naumova E, Nikolich-Zugich J, Pera A, Rector JL, Riddell N, Sanchez-Correa B, Sansoni P, Sauce D, van Lier R, Wang GC, Wills MR, Zieliński M, Pawelec G: CMV and immunosenescence: from basics to clinics. Immun Ageing 2012;9:23.
27 Pawelec G, Ferguson FG, Wikby A: The SENIEUR protocol after 16 years. Mech Ageing Dev 2001;122: 132–134.
28 Franceschi C, Bonafè M, Valensin S, Olivieri F, De Luca M, Ottaviani E, De Benedictis G: Inflamm-aging. An evolutionary perspective on immunosenescence. Ann NY Acad Sci 2000;908:244–254.
29 Leng SX, Tian X, Matteini A, Li H, Hughes J, Jain A, Walston JD, Fedarko NS: IL-6-independent association of elevated serum neopterin levels with prevalent frailty in community-dwelling older adults. Age Ageing 2011;40:475–481.
30 Matheï C, Vaes B, Wallemacq P, Degryse J: Associations between cytomegalovirus infection and functional impairment and frailty in the BELFRAIL Cohort. J Am Geriatr Soc 2011;59:2201–2208.
31 Bandeen-Roche K, Walston JD, Huang Y, Semba RD, Ferrucci L: Measuring systemic inflammatory regulation in older adults: evidence and utility. Rejuvenation Res 2009;12:403–410.
32 Collerton J, Martin-Ruiz C, Davies K, Hilkens CM, Isaacs J, Kolenda C, Parker C, Dunn M, Catt M, Jagger C, von Zglinicki T, Kirkwood TB: Frailty and the role of inflammation, immunosenescence and cellular ageing in the very old: cross-sectional findings from the Newcastle 85+ Study. Mech Ageing Dev 2012;133:456–466.

33 Leng SX, Xue QL, Tian J, Huang Y, Yeh SH, Fried LP: Associations of neutrophil and monocyte counts with frailty in community-dwelling disabled older women: results from the Women's Health and Aging Studies I. Exp Gerontol 2009;44:511–516.
34 Ferrucci L, Penninx BW, Volpato S, Harris TB, Bandeen-Roche K, Balfour J, Leveille SG, Fried LP, Md JM: Change in muscle strength explains accelerated decline of physical function in older women with high interleukin-6 serum levels. J Am Geriatr Soc 2002;50:1947–1954.
35 Morley JE, Malmstrom TK: Frailty, sarcopenia, and hormones. Endocrinol Metab Clin North Am 2013; 42:391–405.
36 Serviddio G, Romano AD, Greco A, Rollo T, Bellanti F, Altomare E, Vendemiale G: Frailty syndrome is associated with altered circulating redox balance and increased markers of oxidative stress. Int J Immunopathol Pharmacol 2009;22:819–827.
37 Roy CN: Anemia in frailty. Clin Geriatr Med 2011; 27:67–78.
38 Jylhävä J, Nevalainen T, Marttila S, Jylhä M, Hervonen A, Hurme M: Characterization of the role of distinct plasma cell-free DNA species in age-associated inflammation and frailty. Aging Cell 2013;12: 388–397.

Anis Larbi, PhD
Singapore Immunology Network (SIgN), Biopolis
Agency for Science Technology and Research (A*STAR)
Singapore (Singapore)
E-Mail Anis_Larbi@immunol.a-star.edu.sg

Tamas Fulop, MD, PhD
Geriatric Division, Department of Medicine
Research Center on Aging, University of Sherbrooke
CSSS-IUGS, Argyll Site, Norton Pavillon
375, rue Argyll, Sherbrooke, QC J1J3H5 (Canada)
E-Mail Tamas.Fulop@USherbrooke.ca

Theou O, Rockwood K (eds): Frailty in Aging. Biological, Clinical and Social Implications.
Interdiscipl Top Gerontol Geriatr. Basel, Karger, 2015, vol 41, pp 41–53 (DOI: 10.1159/000381161)

Sex Differences in Frailty

Ruth E. Hubbard

Centre for Research in Geriatric Medicine, School of Medicine, The University of Queensland,
Princess Alexandra Hospital, Woolloongabba, Brisbane, Qld., Australia

Abstract

Although women live longer lives than men, they tend to have poorer health status. Here, we review the biological and socio-behavioral factors that may contribute to this sex-frailty paradox. The conceptual framework that frailty is a product of the environment and the recovery rate provides a new understanding of women's frailty burden. Even developed countries may present an environment more adverse for women, and lifestyle factors may increase women's vulnerability to stochastic subcellular events that increase recovery time. The frailty index does not reach the theoretical maximal value of 1; its limit is lower in men (0.61) compared to women (0.69). Perhaps deterministic characteristics omitted in current deficit counts, such as reduced emotional adaptability, are more prevalent in men. Alternatively, different limits may result from quantitative evolutionary design, such as a fitness-frailty pleiotropy in men or fertility-frailty pleiotropy in women. The engineering principle of safety factors (maximal capacity divided by routine functioning) may also be informative. If the human system has the same safety factor as its organs (approximately 2.5), men may be 'calibrated' around a frailty index of 0.244, compared to 0.276 for women. Because 0.25 represents the tipping point between functional independence and reliance on others, evolutionary design may have allowed for some limited dependence in women, perhaps motivated by the perinatal period.

Although women live longer lives than men, they tend to have poorer health. This well-described phenomenon, termed the male-female health-survival paradox [1], is one of several fundamental paradoxes of aging [2]. It could also be conceptualized as a sex-frailty paradox [3]. Compared to their age-matched male peers, women could be considered both more frail (because frailty is intended to be a summary measure of health status) and less frail (because they are less vulnerable to the adverse outcome of death). While for both men and women, increasing frailty is associated with worse mortality, it seems clear than this vulnerability cannot be linked directly to frailty status. Female sex seems to be a mediating factor, but not the only one: smoking and social vulnerability also influence how risk is expressed in relation to frailty.

Here, we update a previous review [3] on the biological, social and behavioral factors that may explain the greater longevity of women. We consider the factors contributing to frailty status, evaluating the reasons why older women have a greater deficit burden. The measurement of frailty by a frailty index is consistent with the conceptualization of aging as the failure of a complex system. We explore how this measurement may afford a mechanistic understanding of the sex-frailty paradox.

Sex Differences in Life Expectancy

In most countries throughout the developed and developing world, women tend to have longer life expectancies at birth and lower age-specific mortality rates. There are a few exceptions; for example, women in some South Asian countries have shorter life expectancies, which is thought to be secondary to the preferential treatment of male children and complications associated with pregnancy and childbirth.

Historical evidence suggests that the longer lifespans of women are not a recent phenomenon. Although some people believe that men lived longer than women in ancient and medieval times, historical documents from northern Italy from as early as the 14th century and from England and Wales from the 16th century report higher average ages at death for women. These data have been confirmed by a robust Scandinavian data set from the 18th century [4].

Current data report significant differences in life expectancy in the UK at birth (78.7 years for men and 83.6 years for women), which persist throughout youth and middle age and are proportionally greatest for the oldest old (5.0 years and 6.4 years for 85-year-old men and women, respectively [5]. While there are no definitive explanations for the favorable mortality profile of women, evolutionary theories as well as biological, social and behavioral factors have been proposed.

Evolutionary Theories

After the age of 50 years, the number of men decreases more rapidly compared with the number of women, but overall, there are slightly fewer women than men (for every 100 men, there are 98.6 women). Perhaps the evolutionary advantage is that higher numbers of men achieve species survival by reproduction, even with 'disinvestment' in their survival after reproducing. However, the male andropause reduces rather than terminates fertility, and men are able to father children at advanced chronological ages. Why does such 'disinvestment' not occur in females, who have an earlier and more abrupt cessation to their fecundity? Post-reproductive life spans may increase when old animals still benefits their younger relatives. Post-reproductive mothers enhance the lifetime reproductive success of their offspring by allowing them to breed earlier, more frequently and more successfully [6]. This differential post-reproductive parental investment is an evolutionary adaptive response, which may be mutable rather than fixed.

Biological Factors

Hormones

Hormones may have a central role in the long life expectancy of women. The tendency for cardiovascular disease to occur 10 years earlier in men than women has been attributed to the favorable impact of estrogen on serum lipid profiles. Women who undergo bilateral oophorectomy before the age of 50 years who have never been treated with estrogen therapy have an increased risk of all-cause mortality, heart disease and stroke [7]. Compared with ovarian conservation, bilateral oophorectomy at the time of hysterectomy for benign disease is associated with decreased risks of breast and ovarian cancer but increased risks of all-cause mortality, fatal and nonfatal coronary heart disease, and lung cancer. A comprehensive review has indicated that no subgroup analysis or age group has been found with an association between oophorectomy and increased survival [7]. Increasing age at menopause has been associated with increased survival, even after adjustments for education, smoking, body mass index and marital status [8]. Recent studies have also suggested that estrogen may have protective effects on cerebral areas known to be involved in age-related cognitive functions and Alzheimer's disease [9].

Conversely, testosterone supplementation, even in men with evidence of late-onset hypogonadism, may be associated with a range of adverse effects. Further, the lifespan of male Korean eunuchs was between 14.4 and 19.1 years longer than that of noncastrated men of a similar socio-economic status [10].

Immune System

Women seem to have more robust immune systems and greater resistance to infections throughout their lives, with a slower rate of age-related decline for many immunological parameters. Men tend to experience more severe symptoms and be at increased risk of mortality from a variety of fungal, parasitic and bacterial diseases; these tendencies are exemplified by their response to respiratory infections [11]. Testosterone has been implicated as a cause of immunosuppression, although this finding is controversial [3].

Genetics

Within any species, the sex with heterogametic sex chromosomes (be it male or female) tends to live for a shorter period of time. In women, the presence of two X chromosomes with different potentials may provide a genetic longevity advantage. With increasing chronological age, X chromosome inactivation becomes progressively more skewed toward a predominant single cell line, suggesting inactivation of cell line is disadvantageous to aging [12]. Loci on the X chromosome are protected in the germ line (they spend two-thirds of their time in oocytes rather than in sperm cells, which may account for their slower mutation rates) but are vulnerable in the soma (because only one X chromosome is active in each human female cell, they lack a partner for repair by homologous recombination). Thus, the X chromosome is theoretically attractive as a site of crucial longevity genes, representing a trade-off between germ line propagation and somatic maintenance.

Telomeres have also been implicated in sex longevity differences. Telomere length has long been associated with life span. Adult females have longer telomeres, and because telomeres shorten with each replication, men are more vulnerable to telomere attrition [12]. Even so, telomeres do not appear to be associated with deficit accumulation [13].

Social and Behavioral Factors

Risk Avoidance

Gender-typical risk avoidance behaviors may be central to the longer life expectancy of women. Testosterone seems to have both organizational and activational effects on risk-sensitive financial decisions. Individuals with high testosterone levels are more likely to choose risky careers in finance [14]. In addition, because the administration of testosterone causes men to behave antisocially [15], they are more likely to expose themselves to risks. Women are less likely than men to take psychoactive substances, smoke cigarettes, drink excess alcohol, engage in risky sexual behaviors, take part in hazardous leisure pursuits (e.g. driving too fast) and revert to openly aggressive problem-solving strategies, such as war or suicide. Whether these behavioral differences are a social construct (determined by traditional role expectations) or biologically driven (women's cautiousness secondary to their responsibility for child-rearing) remains controversial. Equal opportunities between the sexes that are currently supported by new policies worldwide may already have impacted the risk exposures of the two sexes, thereby narrowing the difference in life expectancy between the genders.

Health Care Utilization

Significant differences in health care utilization may contribute to women's longevity. Even after adjusting for sex-specific conditions, such as pregnancy, women have a significantly higher mean number of visits to primary care and diagnostic clinics. The sex differences in the utilization of health care services by older people are predominantly explained by their increased number of chronic diseases and reduced health-related quality of life. Interestingly, when specific symptoms, such as back pain and headache, are more closely interrogated, the evidence for greater consultation among women is weak and inconsistent.

Men are less compliant with both prescribed medication and medical advice and tend to delay seeking medical help. The latter has been cited as underpinning men's higher hospitalization and mortality rates.

Nutrition

Women tend to have a higher awareness and better knowledge of nutrition than men. Some 'male' nutritional choices are now known to be associated with adverse outcomes. For example, men are less likely to have breakfast and to take vitamins and supplements and more often eat a less varied diet with more red meat.

These evolutionary, biological, social and behavioral advantages with regard to life expectancy do not translate into advantages with regard to the health status of women. On the contrary, middle-aged and older women have greater levels of disability, more psychological and physical co-morbidities and worse self-rated health, i.e. they accumulate more deficits than men.

Sex Differences in Health Status

The poorer health status of older women has previously been attributed to the impact of their longer life expectancy on age-associated diseases, but it is now known that at any given age, the burden of frailty is greater for women than for men. This is consistent across different frailty measures and across developed and developing countries. These differences in frailty status have been explained by reporting bias, differences in co-morbidities and pathophysiological factors. The conceptualization that accumulated deficits are a product of environmental stresses and recovery time (below) might also provide a mechanistic understanding of health-sex differences.

Reporting Bias

Men and women describe their health statuses according to different aspects of life. Men tend to define their well being through performance and efficiency, whereas women have a more holistic interpretation of health that emphasizes pain and comorbid illness. Men and women with the same functional statuses and comorbidities may therefore report very differently on their self-rated health.

Men are more likely to under-report medical conditions, particularly anxiety and depression. It is easy to envisage how this fact could bias the derivation of frailty indices based on self-reported deficits.

Co-Morbidities

Physical Co-Morbidities

Conditions associated with chronic ill health (such as osteoarthritis, stroke and diabetes mellitus) disproportionately affect women. Men, on the other hand, have a higher prevalence of diseases that do not incur a burden of disability, being either immediately fatal (for example, myocardial infarction) or rapidly progressive (such as pancreatic cancer). Testosterone-induced immunosuppression may decrease men's resistance to infection, but it seems to protect against autoimmune disorders. These diseases typically have a major impact on functional status and quality of life without significantly shortening life expectancy.

Psychological Co-Morbidity

The lifetime probability of developing an episode of depression and/or anxiety is significantly higher in women than in men. Psychological co-morbidity has pervasive and perpetuating effects on health, increasing social vulnerability, reducing positive health behaviors, such as exercise, and triggering the prescription of drugs, such as benzodiazepines, known to increase the risks of unintentional injuries and falls.

The poor psychological health of older women may reflect financial inequality or represent a socialization-based cohort effect. The mid-life peak in psychological distress is found only in low-income households [16]. Furthermore, older men and women who have worked for decades in male-dominated environments show no sex differences in anxiety or depression. Addressing women's relative financial disempowerment and encouraging certain instrumental attributes (task-focused thinking, self-confidence, and assertiveness) may be protective to lifelong mental health.

Cognitive Co-Morbidity

The incidence of dementia is higher in women than in men. Proposed pathogenic explanations were initially focused on amyloid deposition; for example, mitochondria seem to be protected against amyloid-beta toxicity in younger but not older females, which is possibly secondary to falling estrogen levels. However, the association between dementia and specific underlying pathological features becomes weaker with age [17], and dementia in older people is increasingly recognized to be associated with poor general health. In one study of 7,239 cognitively intact community dwellers, the incidence of dementia over 10 years of follow-up increased exponentially with an increasing index of accumulated deficits not known to predict dementia [18]. In this context, considering that women have more physical and psychological co-morbidities, it is unsurprising that they also have a higher prevalence of dementia.

Pathophysiological Factors

Inflammation

Evidence is emerging that the pathophysiology of frailty may differ between the sexes. Inflammation, previously implicated in frailty development, may play a more critical role in women. High concentrations of the inflammatory markers C-reactive protein and fibrinogen are more strongly predictive of incident frailty in women than in men [19]. Furthermore, in older women, the association between sarcopenia and lower cognitive functioning seems to be partly due to systemic inflammation [20]. Older women accumulate more abdominal fat than older men, and this may act as a source of low-grade systemic inflammation, contributing to their frailty status.

Other pathways may be more important in men. Levels of adiponectin, an adipokine with anti-inflammatory and insulin-sensitizing properties, are positively correlated with an increasing number of components of frailty in older men but not in women [21]. In men, the risk of frailty increases linearly with decreased testosterone, whereas in women, the relationship between testosterone and frailty is U-shaped [22]. Body habitus may be an important mediator in this regard. The association of free testosterone with frailty is confined to obese women [22]. The complex inter-relationships between adiposity, hormone levels and frailty status should be stratified by sex in further inquiries.

Childbirth

A 'trade-off' between longevity and reproduction was initially proposed by Westendorp and Kirkwood, evidenced by a negative correlation between number of progeny and longevity in historical datasets from the British aristocracy [23]. A similar trade-off has been observed in other species, including fruit flies and birds, and in contemporary female populations in Europe.

It is theoretically possible that women have poorer health in older age because of their physiological investment in reproduction. Childbirth necessitates a high level of physiological investment. The energetic and nutritional demands of pregnancy and breast-feeding render reproductive costs that are much greater in women than in men. Bearing sons may have particularly high physiological costs, due to their faster rates of intrauterine growth and heavier than average birth weights.

Frailty as a Product of the Recovery Rate and the Environment

Queuing theory has recently been used to provide a conceptual framework for the origin of deficit accumulation [24]. Reformulation of Little's law [the average number of items in a queuing system (L) equals the average arrival rate (λ) multiplied by the average waiting time of an item in the system (W)] facilitates consideration of the average number of deficits present in an individual (L) as a product of only the following

2 factors: the rate of environmental stresses (λ) and the average recovery time (W). This framework may provide new perspectives on the tendency of women to accumulate a greater number of deficits than their age-matched male peers.

Environmental Stresses May Affect Women More Than Men

On a macroscopic level, women and men residing at the same geographical location are exposed to the same threats, such as extremes of climate, disease outbreaks and neighborhood deprivation. However, even within the same household, stresses may not be sex-balanced. In other words, even developed countries may present an environment more adverse for women than for men. Socio-economic sex inequalities relating to financial redistribution, recognition and political representation have been extensively documented. Interestingly, in a recent analysis of European countries, frailty-free life expectancy was lower for women than men, but these differences were less marked in Sweden and Denmark [25]. Scandinavian countries are well recognized for their gender-equality policies, particularly in relation to parental leave and childcare.

Women May Have a Slower Recovery Time

Increasing recovery time with age is likely the stochastic (partly random) outcome of multiple subcellular events. Because these events can be secondary to the effects of lifestyle and environmental factors combined with genetic susceptibility, it is easy to postulate how sex may have a critical role. For example, men's higher levels of education and greater participation in physical activity may reduce the frequency of and/or protect against this subcellular damage.

In the clinical setting, there is some evidence that female sex contributes to poor recovery. At 3 months and 12 months post-ischemic stroke, women have greater functional impairments despite equivalent pre-stroke Barthel scores and stroke severities [26]. Sex differences are also observed after coronary artery bypass grafting, with significantly longer post-operative inpatient stays for women compared to men [27].

Why Can Women Better Tolerate Their Health Deficits?

To recap, at any age, women accumulate more deficits than men; however, these deficits are less lethal [as illustrated in figure 1, from reference 28]. Here, we have reviewed evidence regarding the poorer health statuses and longer life expectancies of women and have explored the underlying reasons for each phenomenon. However, these discussions do not address the crux of the sex-frailty paradox; namely, why women are able to tolerate a greater number of heath deficits.

Three explanations for this paradox have recently been proposed [3]. The first consideration is that there may be some factors affecting life expectancy in older people

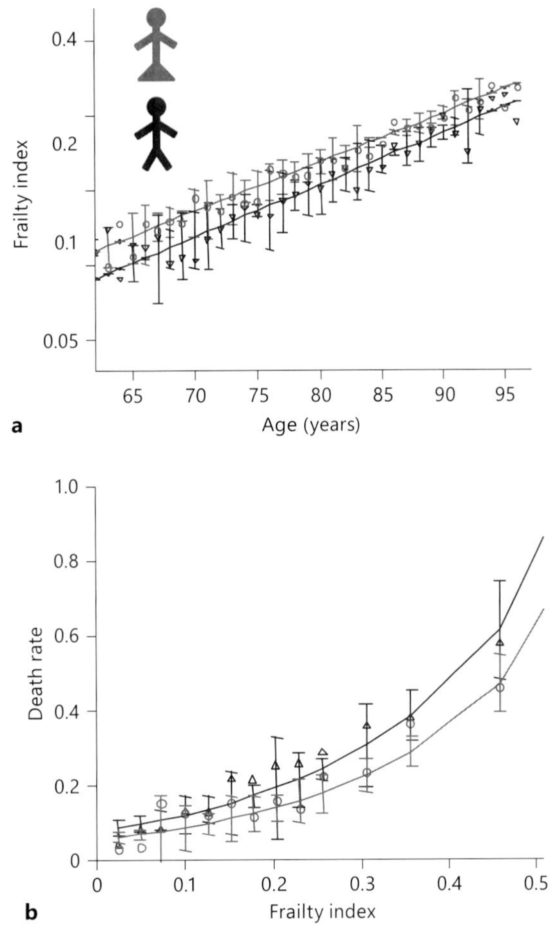

Fig. 1. Sex differences in the relationship between the frailty index and age (**a**) and the frailty index and 3-year mortality (**b**) in men (dark grey lines) and women (light grey lines). The data are from seven population-based community-dwelling samples (n = 33,851). Panel (**b**) data are from the six data sets for which individual mortality data were available (n = 6,427). Source: Mitnitski et al. [28].

that are not captured by current frailty measures and that these factors are present more often in men than in women. The loss of a marital partner, for example, results in relatively greater effects on morbidity and mortality in men compared to women. Less emotional expression and poorer coping mechanisms, which may underpin this observation, are not routinely measured in frailty indices. While growing older can bring wisdom and contentment, in many ways, aging is defined by loss, including bereavements, relinquishment of occupational roles and a decline in physical capabilities. If men are less able to adapt to these losses, they may have more 'hidden' deficits, contributing to their shorter life expectancy.

Recent analyses have reported that the frailty index reaches a lower limit in men (0.61) compared to women (0.69) [29]. This finding raises critical questions regarding quantitative evolutionary design [30]. We can use evolutionary reasoning to understand, in terms of ultimate rather than proximate causation, why the limits to the frailty index have the numerical value that they do, rather than some higher or lower value. The second and third explanations previously proposed for the sex-frailty paradox, namely a male fitness-frailty pleiotropy or a female fertility-frailty pleiotropy, both invoke the concept of quantitative evolutionary design. In the former, older men pay the price for more optimal physiological functioning during youth with a lower threshold for system failure in old age. At any given level of the frailty index, men have changed more from their baseline status compared to women. Because the male system is calibrated differently, older men have lower physiological reserves such that their health deficits are more lethal. Conversely, a female fertility-frailty pleiotropy might be the key driver for greater physiological reserves in women. Childbirth and child rearing necessitate high levels of energetic and nutritional investment; thus, women who have children live shorter lives. The female 'complex system' may be designed for maximum fecundity, with higher levels of frailty among older women but anticipation of equal life expectancies between the sexes. Women currently are limiting the number of children that they bear, and their life expectancies may be longer than predicted by evolutionary design.

Safety Factors and Quantitative Evolutionary Design

Consideration of safety factors is congruent with quantitative evolutionary design and may provide a new perspective on the sex-frailty paradox. In engineering terminology, the safety factor of a structure is its maximal strength (the strength that it is designed to possess) divided by the load that it is expected to routinely bear [31]. This factor is summarized in the following equation:

$$\text{safety factor} = \frac{\text{material strength}}{\text{design load}}.$$

It can also be conceptualized as follows:

$$\text{safety factor} = \frac{\text{maximal capability}}{\text{usual functioning}}.$$

Engineers consider several issues when determining safety factors [30]. The coefficient of variation of load, the coefficient of variation of capacity, deterioration of capacity with time and a high cost of failure are characteristics that would necessitate a higher safety factor. Hence, an external passenger lift that often carries only one person in calm weather but may also carry 10 people in high winds would need a high safety factor (typically of about 12). The cost of initial construction, cost of maintenance, cost of operation and opportunity cost of the occupied space are all considerations that motivate lower safety factors. A dumb waiter does not, therefore, need to have as high of a safety factor as the aforementioned passenger lift (it is usually about 5). Engineered safety factors are higher for buildings made of wood (6), which may deteriorate over time, than for those made of steel (2).

The principle of safety factors has been investigated in human biological and physiological systems [30, 31] by dividing the maximal capability by routine function. In humans, organs tend to have a safety factor of between 2 and 3. The small intestine and lungs, for example, are capable of absorbing nutrients and taking up oxygen, respectively, at twice the rates observed physiologically. Safety factors have also been investigated using a slightly different construct by dividing normal function by adequate function. Again, safety factors of between 2 and 3 have been reported. For myocardial oxygen consumption, vision and hearing, approximately 33% of normal function represents a threshold value for failure [32] (safety factor = 3). Resection studies of the human liver and small bowel have shown that survival is difficult for patients who have lost half of their original organ mass [30] (safety factor = 2).

Applying the principle of scaling [33], the characteristics of organs are likely to manifest at the level of the whole system. We therefore hypothesize here that the safety factor of humans is 2.5. In the formula equating safety factors to a system's maximal capability divided by its usual functioning, the maximal capability of the male system could be considered to be 0.61 (its frailty index limit) and that of the female system to be 0.69 [29]. Hence, the male system is designed around a frailty index score of 0.244, compared to 0.276 for the female system.

A frailty index of 0.25 has been mooted as the cut-off between fitness and frailty in community-dwelling older people [34]. When frailty index scores were contextualized with clinical descriptors, a mean score of 0.22 denoted those who were 'apparently vulnerable – although not frankly dependent, these people commonly complain of being slowed up or have disease symptoms', while 0.27 described those who were 'mildly frail – with limited dependence on others for instrumental activities of daily living' [35]. A frailty index score of 0.25 seems to represent a 'tipping point' from functional independence to dependence on others. In terms of evolutionary design, 'usual functioning' for both men and women may be focused on independence. This hypothesis resonates with numerous qualitative studies reporting that both men and women prioritize maintenance or return of independence above any other goals. Acquisition of knowledge, appreciation of beauty and love of family may be less critical attributes. While the male system is designed around absolute functional independence, 'usual functioning' for women enables some limited dependence on others. This design may be advantageous from an evolutionary perspective, allowing some assistance during perinatal periods.

The hypothesis that survival for both men and women is calibrated around a state of functional independence does not denigrate any people who are born or become dependent. On the contrary, quantitative evolutionary design suggests that the maximal value has been set at a level that the system as a whole can support.

Conclusions

In old age, women are both frailer, with poorer health status, and more robust, with longer life spans. While some factors contributing to these phenomena (such as genetics) are fixed, others (particularly social and behavioral factors) are mutable, and sex-frailty may become a less significant paradox in future cohorts. On the other hand, quantitative evolutionary design may underpin the frailty burden of women, and ultimate causation will be less amenable to intervention. The sex-frailty paradox raises fundamental questions regarding the etiology, manifestations and management of frailty. Studies of frailty index behaviors according to sex and across different cultures and environments are therefore the focus of further inquiries by our group.

Acknowledgments

I would like to thank Ana Koleva-Thompson from the Department of Primary Care and Public Health, Cardiff University, for her thoughtful comments on an earlier version of the manuscript.

References

1 Oksuzyan A, Juel K, Vaupel JW, Christensen K: Men: good health and high mortality. Sex differences in health and aging. Aging Clin Exp Res 2008;20:91–102.
2 Blagosklonny MV: Paradoxes of aging. Cell Cycle 2007;6:2997–3003.
3 Hubbard RE, Rockwood K: Frailty in older women. Maturitas 2011;69:203–207.
4 Gage TB: Are modern environments really bad for us? Revisiting the demographic and epidemiologic transitions. Am J Phys Anthropol 2005;S41:96–117.
5 United Nations: Population ageing and development: ten years after Madrid. United Nations, Department of Economic and Social Affairs, Population Division, 2012.
6 Lahdenpera M, Lummaa V, Helle S, Tremblay M, Russell AF: Fitness benefits of prolonged post-reproductive lifespan in women. Nature 2004;428:178–181.
7 Parker WH, Broder MS, Chang E, Feskanich D, Farquhar C, Liu Z, Shoupe D, Berek JS, Hankinson S, Manson JE: Ovarian conservation at the time of hysterectomy and long-term health outcomes in the nurses' health study. Obstet Gynecol 2009;113:1027–1037.
8 Yonker JA, Chang V, Roetker NS, Hauser TS, Hauser RM, Atwood CS: Hypothalamic-pituitary-gonadal axis homeostasis predicts longevity. Age (Dordr) 2013;35:129–138.
9 Lord C, Engert V, Lupien SJ, Pruessner JC: Effect of sex and estrogen therapy on the aging brain: a voxel-based morphometry study. Menopause 2010;17:846–851.
10 Min KJ, Lee CK, Park HN: The lifespan of Korean eunuchs. Curr Biol 2012;22:R792–R793.
11 Falagas ME, Mourtzoukou EG, Vardakas KZ: Sex differences in the incidence and severity of respiratory tract infections. Respir Med 2007;101:1845–1863.
12 Seifarth JE, McGowan CL, Milne KJ: Sex and life expectancy. Gend Med 2012;9:390–401.
13 Collerton J, Martin-Ruiz C, Davies K, Hilkens CM, Isaacs J, Kolenda C, Parker C, Dunn M, Catt M, Jagger C, von Zglinicki T, Kirkwood TB: Frailty and the role of inflammation, immunosenescence and cellular ageing in the very old: cross-sectional findings from the Newcastle 85+ Study. Mech Ageing Dev 2012;133:456–466.
14 Sapienza P, Zingales L, Maestripieri D: Gender differences in financial risk aversion and career choices are affected by testosterone. Proc Natl Acad Sci U S A 2009;106:15268–15273.
15 Zak PJ, Kurzban R, Ahmadi S, Swerdloff RS, Park J, Efremidze L, Redwine K, Morgan K, Matzner W: Testosterone administration decreases generosity in the ultimatum game. PLoS One 2009;4:e8330.

16 Lang IA, Llewellyn DJ, Hubbard RE, Langa KM, Melzer D: Income and the midlife peak in common mental disorder prevalence. Psychol Med 2011;41: 1365–1372.
17 Savva GM, Wharton SB, Ince PG, Forster G, Matthews FE, Brayne C; Medical Research Council Cognitive Function and Ageing Study: Age, neuropathology, and dementia. N Engl J Med 2009;360: 2302–2309.
18 Song X, Mitnitski A, Rockwood K: Nontraditional risk factors combine to predict Alzheimer disease and dementia. Neurology 2011;77:227–234.
19 Gale CR, Baylis D, Cooper C, Sayer AA: Inflammatory markers and incident frailty in men and women: the English Longitudinal Study of Ageing. Age (Dordr) 2013;35:2493–2501.
20 Canon ME, Crimmins EM: Sex differences in the association between muscle quality, inflammatory markers, and cognitive decline. J Nutr Health Aging 2011;15:695–698.
21 Tsai JS, Wu CH, Chen SC, Huang KC, Chen CY, Chang CI, Chuang LM, Chen CY: Plasma adiponectin levels correlate positively with an increasing number of components of frailty in male elders. PLoS One 2013;8:e56250.
22 Carcaillon L, Blanco C, Alonso-Bouzón C, Alfaro-Acha A, Garcia-García FJ, Rodriguez-Mañas L: Sex differences in the association between serum levels of testosterone and frailty in an elderly population: the Toledo Study for Healthy Aging. PLoS One 2012; 7:e32401.
23 Westendorp RG, Kirkwood TB: Human longevity at the cost of reproductive success. Nature 1998;396: 743–746.
24 Mitnitski A, Song X, Rockwood K: Assessing biological aging: the origin of deficit accumulation. Biogerontology 2013;4:709–717.
25 Romero-Ortuno R, Fouweather T, Jagger C: Cross-national disparities in sex differences in life expectancy with and without frailty. Age Ageing 2014;43: 222–228.
26 Knauft W, Chhabra J, McCullough LD: Emergency department arrival times, treatment, and functional recovery in women with acute ischemic stroke. J Womens Health (Larchmt) 2010;19:681–688.
27 Ott RA, Gutfinger DE, Alimadadian H, Selvan A, Miller M, Tanner T, Hlapcich WL, Gazzaniga AB: Conventional coronary artery bypass grafting: why women take longer to recover. J Cardiovasc Surg (Torino) 2001;42:311–315.
28 Mitnitski A, Song X, Skoog I, Broe GA, Cox JL, Grunfeld E, Rockwood K: Relative fitness and frailty of elderly men and women in developed countries and their relationship with mortality. J Am Geriatr Soc 2005;53:2184–2189.
29 Shi J, Yang Z, Song X, Yu P, Fang X, Tang Z, Peng D, Mitnitski A, Rockwood K: Sex differences in the limit to deficit accumulation in late middle-aged and older Chinese people: results from the Beijing Longitudinal Study of Aging. J Gerontol A Biol Sci Med Sci 2014;69:702–709.
30 Diamond J: Quantitative evolutionary design. J Physiol 2002;542(Pt 2):337–345.
31 Alexander RM: A theory of mixed chains applied to safety factors in biological systems. J Theor Biol 1997;184:247–252.
32 Bortz WM 2nd: A conceptual framework of frailty: a review. J Gerontol A Biol Med Sci 2002;57:M283–M288.
33 Howlett SE, Rockwood K: New horizons in frailty: ageing and the deficit-scaling problem. Age Ageing 2013;42:416–423.
34 Rockwood K, Andrew M, Mitnitski A: A comparison of two approaches to measuring frailty in elderly people. J Gerontol A Biol Sci Med Sci 2007;62:738–743.
35 Rockwood K, Song X, MacKnight C, Bergman H, Hogan DB, McDowell I, Mitnitski A: A global clinical measure of fitness and frailty in elderly people. CMAJ 2005;173:489–495.

Ruth E. Hubbard
Centre for Research in Geriatric Medicine, School of Medicine
The University of Queensland, Princess Alexandra Hospital
Woolloongabba, Brisbane, QLD 4102 (Australia)
E-Mail r.hubbard1@uq.edu.au

Theou O, Rockwood K (eds): Frailty in Aging. Biological, Clinical and Social Implications.
Interdiscipl Top Gerontol Geriatr. Basel, Karger, 2015, vol 41, pp 54–65 (DOI: 10.1159/000381162)

Frailty and the Microbiome

Conor J. Meehan[a, b] · Morgan G.I. Langille[a, c] · Robert G. Beiko[a]

[a]Faculty of Computer Science, [b]Department of Biochemistry and Molecular Biology and [c]Department of Pharmacology, Dalhousie University, Halifax, N.S., Canada

Abstract

From the moment of birth, the human body plays host to a rich diversity of microbes. Body sites such as the skin, the gut and the mouth support communities of microorganisms (collectively known as the *microbiome*) that are both numerous and diverse. As our understanding of the microbiome advances, it is evident that these microbial populations participate in a multitude of symbiotic associations with us. The disruption of these associations can lead to a range of diseases beyond mere pathogenesis as microbial nutrition, signaling, and immune defense break down. It is known that changes in microbial composition occur as the human host ages and that diet and living conditions influence the microbiome of older individuals. However, the link between the microbiome and frailty is as yet mostly unexplored. Although the microbiome is likely to influence health factors that contribute to frailty, further work is needed to determine whether overall microbial signatures of frailty exist and, if so, what the diagnostic and therapeutic utility of these signatures might be.

Our Resident Microbes: Numerous, Diverse and Differentiated

The human microbiome is a collective term that was coined in the year 2000 to refer to all microbes that reside within and on the human body. There are an estimated 10^{14} microbial cells associated with a typical human host, a figure ten times greater than the number of human cells. Although often referred to as a singular entity, the 'human microbiome' in fact comprises many distinct microbial populations that dwell in different body sites such as the skin, the mouth, the airways, the gut and the vagina. It is also proposed that microbial communities reside in sites once thought to be sterile such as the blood, the brain and the lower respiratory tract.

Different body sites typically contain highly distinct sets of microorganisms due to differences in nutrient availability, pH, oxygen, and host-derived factors such as immune responses. Only a small handful of microbial taxa such as *Staphylococcus* are detectable in all body sites, but even these few taxa are not found in all sampled individuals and, when found, differ greatly in their relative abundance [1]. Individual body sites are often dominated by specific genera in the majority of healthy individuals. For instance, the gut microbiome is primarily composed of genera such as *Bacteroides, Faecalibacterium* and *Eubacterium*, whereas the oral microbiome is dominated by *Prevotella*, *Neisseria* and *Veillonella* [1]. Although much of the effort to date in characterizing the human microbiome has focused on prokaryotes (Bacteria and, to a lesser extent, Archaea), the human microbiome also comprises a multitude of viruses, most of which infect bacteria, and eukaryotes, especially fungi such as *Candida* and *Ascomycota*, and protists such as *Blastocystis* [2]. In this review, we will focus on the bacterial component of the microbiome, particularly the human gut microbiome since it has been the most intensively studied and has been the focus in many studies of human health to date.

Different body sites clearly have different sets of associated microbes. Still, the variation within a single body site can be very high. For example, over 1,000 different species have been linked to the adult human gut microbiome, most of which are drawn from a small number of bacterial groups (notably classes Clostridia and Bacteroidia). Individuals harbor only a small subset of these species in their gut at any given time, typically ~150, and samples from different individuals often differ greatly in the bacteria that are present [3]. Even more striking than individual-to-individual variation is the degree to which the species-level composition of an individual's microbiome can change in a matter of weeks or even days. An early demonstration of this variability was the study by Caporaso et al. [4], which sampled the microbiota from the gut, the tongue and the palms of two subjects nearly every day for over a year. They demonstrated clear separation between body sites in terms of microbial composition, but often, no core set of species was present at every time point within a body site. Instead, they postulated that two temporal community types existed: a persistent set that was present for extended periods of time and a transient set that appeared in short bursts. Within a body site, these two communities are often drawn from distinct sets of genera, but they often share similar higher taxonomic ranks such as phylum and class. Although specific species are not always present in different individuals or even at different times within a host, related species are often found within specific body sites for all individuals.

Although much remains to be learned about the factors that shape the composition of our microbiota at different body sites, it is already clear that the host environment plays a key role and that fluctuations in the host environment can lead to rapid alterations in the microbiome.

Diet is a prominent influence on the composition of the gut microbiome, with large differences observed between agrarian and 'Western' diets [5]. In one study, a set of germ-free *(gnotobiotic)* mice were inoculated with the same set of microbes, after which all mice were placed on a low fat, plant-based diet (agrarian diet). One month later, half of the mice were switched to a high fat, high sugar diet (Western diet). A shift in the gut microbiome composition was evident after a single day on the Western diet, and the microbiomes of these mice reached a new equilibrium after 7 days. This shift was primarily in the form of an increase in members of the Firmicute classes Erysipelotrichi and Bacilli and a decrease in the proportion of Bacteroidetes [5]. These diet-induced differences were also observed between fecal samples collected from humans in Malawi and the United States [6]. Such host environment-induced changes have also been observed in other body sites.

In addition to diet, other lifestyle factors are associated with changes in the microbiome. Delima et al. [7] examined the effects of smoking on the oral microbiome and associated diseases. Smoking is often linked to the onset of chronic periodontitis (inflammation of the tooth-associated tissue), and the study authors observed an increase in the pathogenic bacteria that cause periodontitis, which were selectively favored in smokers [7]. This switch in the microbiome from a healthy to a diseased state can be reversed through the cessation of smoking [7], thus demonstrating the critical link between host-derived environmental factors and microbiome composition, which, in turn, can feed back into specific disease states within the host.

An individual's genetic makeup can also influence the composition of their microbiome. Twins have often been shown to have more similar microbiomes than unrelated individuals, although this may be due to cohabitation influences such as environmental interactions and diet [6]. Variations in individual host genes have been associated with changes in the microbiome. One such gene, *MEFV*, encodes pyrin, which is involved in inflammation, and genetic variants of *MEFV* have been linked to changes in microbial community composition [8]. Similar links have been observed between other human genes and microbiome constituents. Such genes are often part of the immune system (e.g. encoding receptors or lysozymes) or metabolism (e.g. encoding leptin) [8]. These and many other examples illustrate the plasticity of the human microbiome, in which shifts in microbiome composition are influenced by both the human and external environments.

Key Functions of the Human Microbiome

If the bacteria and other microorganisms that constitute our microbiome were simply passengers that contributed little to our overall health, then there would be limited clinical interest in understanding our resident microbiota. However, it is increasingly evident that we and our microbes interact in a multitude of ways; in many cases, these interactions are symbiotic, beneficial to both the human host and the resident microbes. It is also evident that the removal of some of these key functions can have serious negative consequences on the host, leading to a state known as *dysbiosis* in which this normal symbiotic association is disrupted.

Key factors specific to the human gut microbiome include adhesins, which facilitate attachment to host cells and other surfaces, and sugar-harvesting complexes, which are essential for the uptake of key sources of energy. Although investigations of the genes present in the human microbiome have discovered these and other important functions, the majority of genes linked to environmental adaptation do not have any known function [3]. Establishing the functions of these genes using experimental and computational approaches is an active area of research.

In addition to the functions that allow microbes to reside within the human GI tract, the microbiome performs a multitude of functions for the human host. Many microorganisms ferment sugars into short-chain fatty acids (SCFAs), which are subsequently absorbed by the surrounding epithelial cells. SCFAs such as acetate, propionate and butyrate play many roles in the human body, ranging from muscle function to protection against colon cancer [3, 9]. The gut microbiome also executes metabolic pathways such as amino acid synthesis and vitamin production; many of these products are taken up by the host and used in our own metabolism. Another main function of our resident microbiota is colonization resistance, the exclusion of exogenous pathogenic species through colonization by commensal microbes. Primary commensal bacteria such as members of the family Lachnospiraceae have been shown to exclude highly toxic pathogens such as *Clostridium difficile* through the production of butyrate or by out-competing for nutrients [10]. Through mechanisms like these, our microbiome becomes an extension of both our metabolic and immune systems.

The influence of the microbiome on the human host is not locally restricted to the tissues at the corresponding body site. Systemic effects of the microbiome have been reported involving many different organs, implicating that resident microorganisms both cause and protect from disease. Several interactions between the microbiome and the immune system have been documented, including effects of the microbiome on the complement system, T-cell maturity, inflammation responses and protection from pathogens [11]. These influences can be positive, such as shaping the development of lymphoid structures, or negative, such as inducing a chronic inflammatory response. Other systems are also affected by resident microbiota. Links have been identified between the gut microbiome and behavior in mouse models, suggesting that distant microbial communities impact brain function [12]. Such ties extend to other major organs such as the heart, as well. For example, the metabolism of L-carnitine by the gut microbiota has been linked to an increase in atherosclerosis (thickening of an artery wall due to fatty deposits) through the production of trimethylamine N-oxide [13]. The separation of the microbiome from our own biology is difficult, and many refer to the conglomeration of the microbiome and the host as a 'holobiont'.

The list of crucial functions provided by our microbiome is long and growing. However, how can these functions be consistently provided to the host, given what we know about the extreme variability in the species composition of the human microbiome? To some extent, different microbes are able to provide the same functions, which allows for functional stability even as different species and sets of species increase or decrease in abundance. As a consequence, although variation is often observed in the species composition of the human microbiome, even within the same individual over time, the functional repertoire of the human gut microbiome appears to be more stable. Additionally, shifts in the microbiome may reflect environmental changes such as different stages of human development, alterations in immune states, or changes in nutrient availability. For example, rapid shifts in response to dietary changes (e.g. [5]) may be due to the selection of microbes that are able to digest the nutrients present in the new diet.

From Healthy Communities to Dysbiosis

Although many different types of bacteria can provide the same important functions, some shifts in the composition of the microbiome are associated with the loss of key functions and with the progression to a diseased or dysbiotic state. The clearest such examples occur when a 'healthy' microbiome gives way to pathogens that directly attack the human host. Antibiotic treatments administered against one pathogen affect the entire microbial community, not just the intended target; the consequent sweeping changes to the gut environment can create an opportunity for other pathogens to take hold. *C. difficile* infection is often preceded by antibiotic treatment, which results in the elimination of symbiotic bacteria that compete with *C. difficile* and even directly suppress its growth [10]. *C. difficile* produces several toxins that cause severe inflammation and recurrent diarrhea, leading to dehydration and even toxic megacolon and death. Treatment of *C. difficile* with antibiotics is often ineffective since 'normal' microflora are not restored, and the cycle of microbial dysbiosis perpetuates. As an alternative to the use of harsh, broad-spectrum antibiotics, bacteriotherapy (for example, in the form of a fecal transplant from a healthy individual) is currently being tested to repopulate the human gut with the correct microbes. This use of the microbiome as a therapeutic target and tool highlights the integration between the microbiome and the host and paves the way for future investigations of the effect of dysbiosis on different aspects of the human condition.

Less clear is the emerging picture of subtle shifts in the microbiome that can lead to (or at the very least reflect) disease. The close connection between the gut microbiome and human health is prominent in several ailments such as Crohn's disease, inflammatory bowel disease, type II diabetes, and obesity. Although these associations are not yet fully understood, it appears that many diseases and conditions are associated with dysbiosis. Inflammatory bowel disease was found to be associated with a marked reduction in certain groups of bacteria such as *Lactobacillus* and increases in other groups such as Clostridia [14]. The reduction in SCFAs due to dysbiosis has been postulated to be a cause of diarrhea, while the inflammation associated with many chronic bowel diseases is likely due to changes in signaling between epithelial cells and the gut microbiome [14]. The far-reaching effects of the gut microbiome have also been linked to conditions such as anxiety and depression due to the influence of bacteria on the stress response system [15]. Bacteria entering the gut may trigger specific neuron activation, resulting in both altered gut motility and systemic effects on the hypothalamic-pituitary-adrenal axis. As clinical interest in our microbiomes increases, it is likely that many more connections will be added to this web of cause and effect between resident microbes and human health.

What Role Do Microbes Play in Aging and Frailty?

A strong link has been demonstrated between the composition of the gut microbiome and transitions that occur at different life stages in the human host. Newborn babies are thought to be completely or near sterile at birth, followed by rapid colonization post-delivery. Microbial diversity is initially low and increases rapidly in the first few years of human life [16]. As diversity increases, the composition of the microbiome can shift [16], and the makeup of microbes is different in each infant [6]. Even so, it appears that one genus, *Bifidobacterium*, dominates in the infant gut and then decreases rapidly, although not to complete absence, with maturation [6]. Functionally, the infant gut microbiome is dominated by species that are involved in lactate metabolism and plant polysaccharide breakdown. Upon a shift in diet toward solid food, the microbial composition of the gut also shifts to a state similar to that of adults, in which the gut microbiome is primarily comprised of *Bacteroidetes* and *Clostridia* species and in which SCFA production and vitamin (primarily dietary B12) and carbohydrate metabolism increase [6, 16]. Once a child has reached the age of 3 years, the gut microbiome makeup is generally similar to that of adults [6].

Evidence is emerging that the gut microbiome also changes in the later stages of life, albeit in a less dramatic way than in the infant-to-child transition. Several factors have been suggested to underlie this shift, including reduced speed of intestinal motility and decreased immune system function, resulting in a relaxation of the regulation of bacterial colonization (see [17] for references). Other environmental changes in older populations, such as differences in diet and changes in living conditions, appear to impact the microbiome, as well. A study comparing subjects over the age of 65 (and a small cohort of younger subjects) demonstrated that living conditions had a strong influence on the microbiome [18]. Individuals living in a long-term residential facility had marked differences in their gut microbiome compared to subjects still living within a community. The gut microbiome of the latter clustered with that of younger adult subjects and was dominated by *Coprococcus* and *Roseburia*, whereas that of the former primarily included *Parabacteroides*, *Eubacterium*, *Anaerotruncus*,

Lactonifactor and *Coprobacillus* [18]. All of these genera are classified within the bacterial phylum Firmicutes, but their ecological roles in the gut are still being explored and likely differ. Diet is an obvious source of variation in the microbiome, but other factors such as medication and frailty may play a role, as well. Another study [17] observed further changes in centenarians compared to people 60–80 years of age. Among the sampled microbiomes, the 60–80-year-old cohort was found to be most similar to younger adults, as was seen in the community-living older individuals of the previous study. The centenarians had a shift in their gut microbiome to a prominence of Proteobacteria and Bacilli and a decrease in *Clostridia* [17]. These dominant groups contain many facultative anaerobes and potential 'pathobionts', species that are opportunistic pathogens in the presence of certain factors such as increased inflammation, which is often associated with advanced host age. It is evident that as age increases, changes occur within the microbiome, and these changes may be linked to either causative or correlated inflammatory agents and other factors associated with aging.

Aging and inflammation contribute greatly to the overall frailty of an individual. Frailty is defined in terms of the combined effect of deficits in cognition, affect, mobility, continence and function [19]. The lethality of such deficits can be influenced by many factors, such as lifestyle, overall health status, levels of inflammation, effectiveness of the immune system and, potentially, the microbiome. Links between the microbiome and inflammation have been shown repeatedly (e.g. [14]); the microbiome may also be linked to cognitive functions such as anxiety [15]. SCFAs affect epithelial cell health and gastrointestinal tract function and even protect against certain invasive pathogens and cancers. As humans age, SCFA production by the microbiome goes down [17], and this event may increase the likelihood of several health deficits, thus influencing the overall frailty of the individual. Specific links between frailty and the microbiome have already been proposed. Subjects with high frailty were found to have a decrease in groups such as *Eubacteria*, *Faecalibacterium* and *Lactobacilli* [20]. All of these groups have protective functions, including the production of SCFAs (specifically butyrate) and the positive stimulation of the immune system, within the gut. Thus, their decrease likely has a negative effect on the health of the gut and potentially has more systemic effects. Specifically, the levels of SCFAs within people of high frailty have been shown to be drastically lower than their levels within less frail individuals [18], supporting this link between gut microbiome metabolite production and the frailty of the host. Conversely, members of the *Oscillibacter* and *Alistipes* genera are increased in highly frail individuals [18]. These genera produce some SCFAs but not butyrate, the main beneficial SCFA. These species produce propionate and acetate, which can influence cholesterol levels [9], although no definitive links between these genera and negative effects on the host are currently known.

It would appear from early studies that the gut microbiome could both reflect and influence the frailty of the host. However, elucidating the structure and function of a given microbiome sample or 'the microbiome' in general is challenging, with the choice of analytical technique potentially influencing the results obtained. Although several other body sites outside of the gut have been studied, their potential roles in aging and frailty are even less well understood. As the microbiomes of other body sites are known to influence a host of health deficits, such as vaginal bacteriosis, psoriasis and cystic fibrosis, it is likely that they too will have an influence on the overall frailty of an individual. Finding such links will require in-depth analysis of the microbiome, the host and the interface between the two.

Exploring the Potential Connection between Microbes and Frailty

As we have seen, several studies have shown links between aging and the microbiome. However, determining which associations are the driving factors behind these changes in the microbiome is confounded by several other changes that occur within the aging population. For example, as people get older, their living conditions often change, such as increases in visits to day hospitals or permanent moves to long-term care facilities [18]. Considering that previous studies have shown that the microbiomes of individuals within the same household tend to be more similar [8], this movement leads to a problem with determining if the changes we see in the microbiome are due to physiological effects of aging or, instead, environmental changes. Additionally, shifts in living conditions also coincide with changes in diet, representing yet another confounding factor in determining the relationship between the individual and his or her microbiome. Therefore, experimental design is a crucial factor in linking various aspects of health and disease to the composition and function of the microbiome. Experiments that control for these confounding variables, for example, by comparing individuals within the same living conditions and with similar diets, allow for the more sensitive interpretation of changes in the microbiome due to actual biological changes in response to aging. Along with controlling for these variables, it is necessary to obtain details about the sampled individual that could impact changes in the microbiome. For instance, previous studies have often not collected samples from those who have taken antibiotics within a particular time frame (e.g. the last 6–12 months) since their microbiome may have been disrupted and may not yet have reached a normal state [21]. It is important to note that medications other than antibiotics may also have effects on the microbiome. Until future studies begin to identify what particular medications disturb the microbiome, collecting data about medication use and other environmental changes is a necessary initial step in determining external influences.

Aside from controlling for environmental factors, future studies will benefit from the collection of physiological and genetic information from the microbiome host. This information can be used to determine specific host-microbiome interactions. For instance, a decrease in vitamin B12 biosynthesis genes within elderly microbiomes has been previously reported [22], and this finding suggests a causal interaction between changes in the microbiome and the B12 deficiencies seen in aging populations. Having actual vitamin B12 measurements from blood samples taken along with microbiome samples can help to validate these types of interactions. Other physiological information, such as clinical measurements performed to calculate a frailty index, could also provide new insights into host-microbiome interactions.

Given the challenges of conducting frailty studies in human populations, animal models are an essential complement for the pursuit of the relationship between the microbiome and frailty. Mice have been used extensively in microbiome studies ranging from regular lab strains to germ-free gnotobiotic mice to 'humanized' mice (in which a human microbiome is transplanted into a germ-free mouse) [23]. In addition, frailty measurements have recently been shown to be just as applicable in mice as they are in people [24], suggesting that animal aging models could be a very useful direction for microbiome studies in the future. Animal models also have the benefit of allowing very detailed longitudinal studies, which are not as practical in humans. Considering the lifespan of a mouse is typically 3 years at most, future studies that include samples throughout the life of the same mouse could provide novel insights into the natural progression of the microbiome and its response to aging. These control studies could then be followed up with further experiments to determine the impact of various factors such as diet, exercise, and medication on the aging microbiome at more than a single time point.

After a well-thought-out sampling procedure is designed, the next challenge is to decide on protocols to study the microbiome. The gut microbiome can be sampled in various ways, but the least invasive method is to simply obtain fecal swabs. Microbial DNA from the sample is then extracted using various protocols and prepared for sequencing. Sequencing technology has improved the throughput from a single sequencing run, such that multiple samples can be adequately sequenced at a single time. Methods for sample collection, sample storage, DNA extraction, sequencing, and computational analysis are all important factors and have been shown to influence the resulting data [25]. As long as the protocol is consistent between samples, then the results, even if biased by the method, can be compared in relative terms. Currently, the two main methods for analyzing microbiomes are to sequence a single gene marker or to sequence all of the DNA from the sample, referred to as the metagenome. In single-gene marker studies, the same fragment of a particular gene, such as the 16S ribosomal RNA gene, is amplified and sequenced at a great depth so that the majority or all of the community is sequenced. These single-gene marker studies provide taxonomic information about the different microbes within each sample, and this information can be used to characterize the diversity both within samples (e.g. the total number of different observed taxa) and between samples (e.g. comparing counts and abundances of organisms across samples). Although common, single-marker studies are limited to making comparisons based on 'Who is there?' and cannot address the question 'What are they doing?'; i.e. what potential functions do the microbes contain and how is that related to changes in the host? This metagenomics approach requires greater sequencing depth since the ideal process is to sample all genes from all organisms in the sample, not just a single marker gene. In addition, metagenomic data are considerably more complex since the volume of sequences is larger and since the organism that each sequence originated from is initially unknown. However, metagenomic studies have revealed additional important insights into the microbiome that are not apparent from single-gene marker studies. For example, several functions seem to be differentially abundant within older people, such as a decrease in vitamin B12 biosynthesis genes, butyrate production and glycan degradation. New bioinformatics methods are needed to enable greater exploration of the data and to understand the links between the microbes identified in the sample and the functions that each microbe is performing. In addition, other methods that focus on what genes are actually being expressed by the microbes or what metabolites are being produced, called metatranscriptomics and metametabolomics, respectively, provide other avenues in understanding the microbiome as a community. Although challenging, integrating data about host genetics and phenotypes and developing methods that can model the interactions between and the pathways and metabolites shared between the host and the microbiome will ultimately lead to a more complete understanding of aging and frailty.

Conclusions

Microbiomics as a discipline has great potential to change how we view and treat a range of diseases. Surveys of the microbiome are now being integrated into many clinical studies, leading to a constant expansion of host factors (such as disease, age, living conditions and diet) that are being tested. The knowledge gained thus far is being translated into diagnostic techniques, and in some cases, into interventions such as fecal transplantation. The technological revolutions that enable this research can both help and hinder our ability to understand the messages of the microbiome; with DNA sequencing technologies and analytical tools in a constant state of refinement and flux, generating repeatable results and comparing results across studies can be nearly impossible. Realizing the promise of microbiomics will depend on not only careful experimental design but also the stabilization of methods and analytical tools and better ways to define the types of microbes that are present, the functions that they perform, and the myriad ways in which they interact with us.

How will a deeper understanding of the microbiome enhance our understanding of frailty? Given the intimate associations seen thus far between microbes and a range of environmental factors, it is reasonable to expect that one or more microbial signatures of frailty may exist. These signatures might manifest not as a set of specific genera or functions that are present in frail individuals but rather as a series of deficits in crucial microbial functions that are reduced in abundance in or completely absent from frail individuals. Dysbiosis, viewed in functional terms, could therefore be directly analogous to human frailty: the lack of several key functions may have a similar impact on the host regardless of which specific functions are lacking. Deficits in microbiome functions may be remediable through bacteriotherapy or the supplementation of missing compounds such as vitamins, but the complexity of the human-microbial association makes it difficult to predict the outcomes of such interventions. With new assessments of the relationship between microbes and frailty, the testing of relevant environmental factors, and advances in sequencing and bioinformatic interpretation of the microbiome, we will soon start to learn what happens to the microbial worlds within us as we become older and more frail.

References

1 Costello EK, Lauber CL, Hamady M, Fierer N, Gordon JI, Knight R: Bacterial community variation in human body habitats across space and time. Science 2009;326:1694–1697.

2 Parfrey LW, Walters WA, Knight R: Microbial eukaryotes in the human microbiome: ecology, evolution, and future directions. Front Microbiol 2011;2:153.

3 Qin J, Li R, Raes J, Arumugam M, Burgdorf KS, Manichanh C, et al: A human gut microbial gene catalogue established by metagenomic sequencing. Nature 2010;464:59–65.

4 Caporaso JG, Lauber CL, Costello EK, Berg-Lyons D, Gonzalez A, Stombaugh J, et al: Moving pictures of the human microbiome. Genome Biol 2011;12:R50.

5 Turnbaugh PJ, Ridaura VK, Faith JJ, Rey FE, Knight R, Gordon JI: The effect of diet on the human gut microbiome: a metagenomic analysis in humanized gnotobiotic mice. Sci Transl Med 2009;1:6ra14.

6 Yatsunenko T, Rey FE, Manary MJ, Trehan I, Dominguez-Bello MG, Contreras M, et al: Human gut microbiome viewed across age and geography. Nature 2012;486:222–227.

7 Delima SL, McBride RK, Preshaw PM, Heasman PA, Kumar PS: Response of subgingival bacteria to smoking cessation. J Clin Microbiol 2010;48:2344–2349.

8 Spor A, Koren O, Ley R: Unravelling the effects of the environment and host genotype on the gut microbiome. Nat Rev Microbiol 2011;9:279–290.

9 Wong JMW, de Souza R, Kendall CWC, Emam A, Jenkins DJA: Colonic health: fermentation and short chain fatty acids. J Clin Gastroenterol 2006;40:235–243.

10 Reeves AE, Koenigsknecht MJ, Bergin IL, Young VB: Suppression of *Clostridium difficile* in the gastrointestinal tracts of germfree mice inoculated with a murine isolate from the family Lachnospiraceae. Infect Immun 2012;80:3786–3794.

11 Hooper L V, Littman DR, Macpherson AJ: Interactions between the microbiota and the immune system. Science 2012;336:1268–1273.

12 Cryan JF, O'Mahony SM: The microbiome-gut-brain axis: from bowel to behavior. Neurogastroenterol Motil 2011;23:187–192.

13 Koeth RA, Wang Z, Levison BS, Buffa JA, Org E, Sheehy BT, et al: Intestinal microbiota metabolism of L-carnitine, a nutrient in red meat, promotes atherosclerosis. Nat Med 2013;19:576–585.

14 Simrén M, Barbara G, Flint HJ, Spiegel BMR, Spiller RC, Vanner S, et al: Intestinal microbiota in functional bowel disorders: a Rome foundation report. Gut 2013;62:159–176.

15 Foster JA, McVey Neufeld K-A: Gut-brain axis: how the microbiome influences anxiety and depression. Trends Neurosci 2013;36:305–312.

16 Koenig JE, Spor A, Scalfone N, Fricker AD, Stombaugh J, Knight R, et al: Succession of microbial consortia in the developing infant gut microbiome. Proc Natl Acad Sci U S A 2011;108(suppl):4578–4585.

17 Biagi E, Nylund L, Candela M, Ostan R, Bucci L, Pini E, et al: Through ageing, and beyond: gut microbiota and inflammatory status in seniors and centenarians. PLoS One 2010;5:e10667.

18 Claesson MJ, Jeffery IB, Conde S, Power SE, O'Connor EM, Cusack S, et al: Gut microbiota composition correlates with diet and health in the elderly. Nature 2012;488:178–184.

19 Rockwood K, Mitnitski A: Frailty in relation to the accumulation of deficits. J Gerontol Ser A Biol Sci Med Sci 2007;62:722–727.

20 Van Tongeren SP, Slaets JPJ, Harmsen HJM, Welling GW: Fecal microbiota composition and frailty. Appl Environ Microbiol 2005;71:6438–6442.
21 Relman DA: The human microbiome: ecosystem resilience and health. Nutr Rev 2012;70(suppl 1):S2–S9.
22 Lan Y, Kriete A, Rosen GL: Selecting age-related functional characteristics in the human gut microbiome. Microbiome 2013;1:2.
23 Gootenberg DB, Turnbaugh PJ: Companion animals symposium: humanized animal models of the microbiome. J Anim Sci 2011;89:1531–1537.
24 Whitehead JC, Hildebrand BA, Sun M, Rockwood MR, Rose RA, Rockwood K, et al: A clinical frailty index in aging mice: comparisons with frailty index data in humans. J Gerontol A Biol Sci Med Sci 2014;69:621–632.
25 Lozupone C, Stombaugh J, Gonzalez A, Ackermann G, Wendel D, Vazquez-Baeza Y, et al: Meta-analyses of studies of the human microbiota. Genome Res 2013;23:1704–1714.

Robert G. Beiko
Faculty of Computer Science
Dalhousie University
6050 University Avenue, Halifax, NS B3H 4R2 (Canada)
E-Mail beiko@cs.dal.ca

Theou O, Rockwood K (eds): Frailty in Aging. Biological, Clinical and Social Implications.
Interdiscipl Top Gerontol Geriatr. Basel, Karger, 2015, vol 41, pp 66–73 (DOI: 10.1159/000381164)

Operationalizing Frailty Using the Frailty Phenotype and Deficit Accumulation Approaches

Olga Theou[a] • Jeremy Walston[b] • Kenneth Rockwood[a]

[a]Geriatric Medicine, Faculty of Medicine, Dalhousie University, Halifax, N.S., Canada; [b]Division of Geriatric Medicine and Gerontology, Department of Medicine, Johns Hopkins University, Baltimore, Md., USA

Abstract

In both demographic and clinical studies, frailty is understood as a multidimensional state of increased vulnerability compared with the status of others of the same age. Of the many theoretical definitions of frailty, two are commonly employed: the physical frailty/phenotypic approach and the deficit accumulation approach. The purpose of this chapter is to discuss how frailty is conceptualized and operationalized based on these two approaches.

The term 'frailty' has been used scientifically since at least 1979, when Vaupel et al. [1] employed it to describe variability in life expectancy (hidden heterogeneity). They borrowed the idea of an individual, unobserved susceptibility to death from the actuarial literature to explain why some individuals tend to have a long life. In geriatric medicine, we are more inclined to see frailty as a nonconstant factor that increases with age. It is worth recalling that the notion of frailty in geriatric medicine arose during the era of the controlled clinical trial, when comprehensive geriatric assessment was shown to be most effective when targeting vulnerable older adults. At one point, such people were called the 'targeted elderly', whereas now, these vulnerable older adults are understood as frail. As the concept of frailty has become more readily accepted, a variety of definitions of frailty have emerged; these definitions are currently the focus of debate. Two of the most commonly used approaches to conceptualize and define frailty are the phenotypic approach and the deficit accumulation approach. The phenotypic definition operationalizes frailty as a biological *syndrome*, whereas the deficit accumulation approach sees frailty as a multidimensional risk *state*. Various sets of criteria have been proposed to operationalize frailty by evaluating specific physiological changes and deficits; however, currently, none of the proposed operational definitions of frailty provide a definitive diagnosis [2, 3]. Most operational definitions of frailty specify impairments in mobility, balance, muscle strength, motor processing, physical function, disability, cognition, nutrition, endurance, and physical activity [2]. Those impairments most commonly specified are physical function, mobility, disability, and cognition [2].

The Deficit Accumulation, or Frailty Index, Approach

This approach sees frailty as a multidimensional risk *state* that can be measured by the quantity rather than by the nature of health problems. Frailty reflects a stochastic dynamic process in a system with high redundancy of multiple interdependent items. On average, this system accumulates deficits that impair the ability of the system to repair damage that arises either externally or as the byproduct of internal processes (e.g. metabolism, respiration, and inflammation), including genetically induced damage. Even though some events can accelerate the development of frailty, typically frailty develops slowly, even insidiously, and this process can vary in important ways between individuals. The deficit accumulation/frailty-as-a-state approach proposes that frail older adults have many things wrong with them; the more things that they have wrong, the higher the likelihood that they will be frail and the greater their risk of adverse health outcomes.

The origin of deficit accumulation can generally be understood from a stochastic point of view. Accordingly, there is a simple relationship between the average number of deficits (N) present in an individual of a certain age, the intensity of the stream of environmental stresses (λ) and the average recovery time (R) [4], which is written as $N = \lambda R$, known as Little's Law in the operation research area [5]. During the individual's life course, both environmental stresses and the recovery time are clearly stochastic (as evidenced by the generally irregular individual trajectories of the frailty index) [6]. In contrast, the population-based trajectories of frailty are clearly regular, showing an acceleration in deficit accumulation that is well fitted by an exponential curve with an exponent of about 0.03. Because the frailty index increases by 10-fold on average between 20 and 90 years of age and because environmental intensity remains on average unchanged, we can conclude from Little's Law that the recovery time is what changes over the life course, explaining the increases in the frailty index value [4].

Operationalizing the Deficit Accumulation Approach

The application of the deficit accumulation approach is the frailty index [7]. This index can include deficits such as symptoms, signs, diseases, disabilities, and laboratory abnormalities. These deficits should be age-related, should be associated with adverse outcomes, and, when combined, should cover several organ systems. Five or 10 specific deficits might not capture all aspects of frailty, which has hindered agreement between investigators on one frailty scale that includes specific deficits. Older adults are very heterogeneous and become frail through different pathways, and any scale that includes enough items could be used as an indicator of frailty, especially if the items are integrated variables such as mobility and physical activity. Prior studies suggest that at least 20 deficits should be considered; 30 or more is preferred to achieve stable estimates [8]. An individual's frailty index score is calculated based on the number of deficits a person has in relation to the total number of measures included in the index (e.g. someone with 10 deficits out of 40 counted has a frailty index of 10/40 = 0.25). In this way, the frailty index score is continuous (0–1); the higher the score, the more likely that the individual is vulnerable to adverse health outcomes.

The population-based studies that have used the frailty index approach (but differing frailty indices, depending on the data available) give robust results: people accumulate an average of 0.03 deficits per year after the age of 70; the frailty index has a strong association with adverse health outcomes; women accumulate more deficits than men of the same age; and the frailty index has maximal limit of approximately 0.7 [8]. These studies, including studies in North America [9], Europe [10], and Australia [11], have all identified nonlinear increases with age. While the relationship between age and frailty index scores generally was best fit with an exponential function (accelerating with age), the relationship between the frailty index score and mortality rate best fit with a sigmoidal (dose-response) function. The sigmoidal relationship between age and mortality in cross-sectional data, which is characterized by an initial acceleration in mortality risk followed by a deceleration at older ages, has been well described in the literature, representing a fundamental observation in the reliability theory of aging.

The existence of a health-survival paradox between genders, in which two people of the same frailty score but different genders demonstrate differing vulnerability (described in detail in Chapter 4), underscores the notion that frailty scales are imperfect in their ability to measure variable risk of death. Other factors beyond gender have been found to influence the relationship between a score on a frailty scale and the risk for mortality, including individual-level factors like social vulnerability, exercise, and tobacco use as well as environmental factors including country of residence. Differing vulnerability at the same level of identified frailty is important consideration because the concept of frailty was initially developed in order to grade this vulnerability itself. This discrepancy suggests that some factors that modify the effect of frailty or that are unmeasured sources of differential vulnerability among people of the same frailty score need to be considered when examining frailty.

The Frailty Phenotype, or Syndromic, Approach

This approach is based on a cluster of signs and symptoms that commonly occur in vulnerable older adults, including weight loss, weakness, fatigue, slowness in walking, and low levels of physical activity. Aggregations of common signs and symptoms have

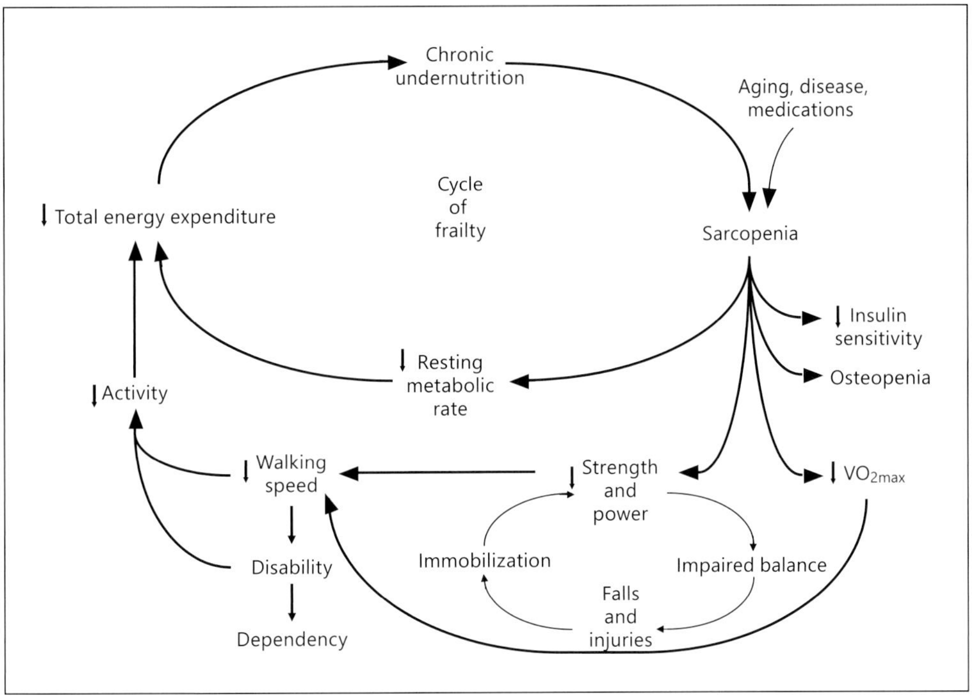

Fig. 1. The cycle of frailty.

long been used in early stages of disease characterization to conceptualize and define medical conditions including type 2 diabetes mellitus, hyperlipidemia, and rheumatological conditions such as lupus. Hence, the conceptualization of frailty as a syndrome with an underlying age-related biological basis was further developed by Fried and Walston [12]. *The Cycle of Frailty*, first published in 1998, facilitated the conceptualization of frailty as a deeply biological entity that largely drives the accumulation of associated adverse outcomes. It also provided an important framework that helped in the development of testable biological hypotheses related to syndromic frailty. This model highlights individual components of a cycle of decline that are associated in a step-wise fashion with other declines, providing the biological basis for the development of vulnerability to functional decline, disease states, and, ultimately, mortality. This model connects the underlying physiology of low energy expenditure, low physical activity, nutritional deficits, and loss of skeletal muscle (sarcopenia) into a cycle of decline (fig. 1). These interconnected domains reinforce each other, and in turn, this interaction influences other crucial physiological systems, including insulin sensitivity, VO_{2max}, muscle strength, and power. These changes then contribute to a subcycle of disability, functional decline, and reduced activity levels that further reinforces the physiological decline. Importantly, this model also suggests multiple possible entry points into an underlying biological cycle of decline and illustrates how specific illnesses, injuries, or medications can trigger and/or accelerate this biological decline. As discussed in Chapter 1, the notion of frailty arising in an interconnected web of deficits can also be seen as consistent with how deficit accumulation accelerates. As noted in that chapter, in a constant environment, the accumulation of deficits is seen to reflect a prolongation of the recovery time.

For example, it is clear that many common chronic disease states, including metastatic or advanced cancers, chronic congestive heart failure, chronic obstructive pulmonary disease, and inflammatory conditions such as rheumatoid arthritis, can help trigger or accelerate the biological cycle of decline that underlies syndromic frailty. However, frailty often exists independently of identifiable disease states. This can be read as further supporting the concept of an independent underlying pathophysiological etiology that is driving syndromic frailty and related outcomes [13]. This pathophysiological change may in part be driven by specific cellular aging processes such as mitochondrial decline and cellular senescence, which contribute to adverse health outcomes in this and the deficit accumulation conceptualizations of frailty.

Operationalizing Phenotypic Frailty

Building on clinical observations of vulnerable older adults, multiple syndromic models of frailty have been developed using data derived from large longitudinal population-based studies of older adults that most often include measures related to clinical observations of vulnerable older adults including weight decline, muscle strength, walking speed and subjective measures of energy levels and physical activity. Early focused efforts in this area include a study by Chin et al. [14] that compared three previously developed working definitions of frailty, namely inactivity combined with (1) low energy intake, (2) weight loss, or (3) low body mass index. The combination of inactivity with weight loss was found to be most strongly associated with reductions in subjective health and performance measures and with increased disease and disability. In addition, the 3-year relative risk for mortality was substantially higher in this group compared to others in the study cohort (odds ratio 4.1, 95% confidence interval 1.8–9.4) [14]. Fried et al. [13] utilized a syndromic approach and developed and operationalized a frailty phenotype based on common physiological signs and symptoms characteristic of frail, older adults. This tool consists of five items, including muscle strength (lowest quartile as determined by dynamometric measurement of grip strength), weight loss (more than 10 pounds of unintended weight loss in the previous year), walking speed (lowest quartile of performance on a timed 15 meter walk), low levels of physical activity as measured by the Minnesota Leisure Time Activities questionnaire, and fatigue (measured by questions about energy levels from a depression survey). It was first operationalized in the Cardiovascular Health Study (CHS), an epidemiological study of over 5,000 community-dwelling adults over the age of 65, who were followed for 9 years in order to better characterize cardiovascular disease and functional decline late in life. The participants were deemed frail if they met three of the five criteria, intermediate, or 'pre-frail', if they met one or two of the criteria, and robust, or not frail, if they met none of the criteria. Seven percent of these

CHS participants met the criteria to be considered as frail at their baseline exam. A significant overlap between disability, chronic illness, and frailty was observed, although there were many frail participants who were not disabled and who did not have medical illnesses, supporting the previously mentioned hypothesis that syndromic or physical frailty has an underlying etiology that is likely independent of disease and disability [13]. Predictive validity analyses were also performed, revealing that those who were frail were significantly more likely to fall, enter a nursing home, be hospitalized, and suffer mortality over 7 years of follow-up. These results have been confirmed in many large cohort studies, including the Women's Health and Aging Study, which demonstrated an even stronger association between frailty and the 3-year mortality rates [15]. This syndromic tool to measure frailty has gone on to become among the most commonly cited frailty measurement tools in the medical literature and has been utilized extensively to assess clinical risk in a variety of settings and to study the biological basis of frailty, chronic disease states, and late-life vulnerability. This syndromic approach to frailty measurement has also been adapted and altered by many investigators in order to more feasibly measure frailty in populations of older adults and in clinical practice. Published validity data for many of these adaptations suggests that these adapted tools also predict adverse outcome in older adults relatively well [16–19]. Future studies in this area are needed to more fully explore the validity of these tools.

To date, the majority of biological studies of frailty have taken place using the syndromic definition of frailty. These studies, which have been carried out as large epidemiological data studies or smaller scale clinical observational studies [20–23], have enabled the identification of core biological changes that are highly related to and perhaps drive the development of frailty and late-life vulnerability to adverse health outcomes observed among frail individuals. Important findings include significant relationships between chronic activation of inflammation as measured by serum cytokine levels, increased hypothalamic-pituitary-adrenal axis activation as measured by salivary cortisol levels, altered glucose metabolism, and decreased mitochondrial mass as key correlates and perhaps drivers of syndromic frailty and its incumbent risk [20–23].

Other Operational Definitions of Frailty

In addition to the frailty phenotype and the frailty index, other operational definitions of frailty include the Edmonton Frail Scale, the Groningen Frailty Indicator, the Tilburg Frailty Indicator, and the 'FRAIL' scale. The Edmonton Frail Scale considers 17 specific deficits, including cognition, general health status, functional independence, social support, medication use, nutrition, mood, continence, and functional performance [24]. The Groningen Frailty Indicator includes measures of physical (including mobility, physical fitness, vision, hearing, nourishment, and polypharmacy), cognitive, and psychosocial health, for a score calculated from 15 items [25]. The Tilburg

Frailty Indicator scores 15 deficits in physical (weight loss, overall physical health, difficulty in walking, balance, vision problems, hearing problems, hand strength, and tiredness), psychological (cognition, depressive symptoms, anxiety, and coping), and social domains (living alone, social relations, and social support) [26]. The FRAIL scale considers five health deficits, forming its acronym: fatigue, resistance, ambulation, illness, and loss of weight; four of these components were obviously taken from the frailty phenotype [27]. New scales are also being proposed: of 27 frailty scales that have been applied to population-based studies, 14 have yet to be used by researchers beyond the group that first proposed them [28]. At the 2012 meeting of the Gerontological Society of America, 13 further frailty scales were newly introduced [29]. When eight frailty scales were recently applied to a representative sample of middle-aged and older Europeans in the Survey of Health, Ageing, and Retirement in Europe (SHARE), they all identified frailty and predicted all-cause mortality, even though they captured related but distinct components and varied in the accuracy of their mortality prediction [30]. Similarly, when three frailty scales were compared in the European Male Ageing Study, they showed differing ability to predict mortality [31]. Many of these scales have been developed to meet the needs of specific research studies and have not been operationalized in other populations. Compared with the more focused effort of the frailty phenotype, the broad heterogeneity in measurement domains and in the specific measurements contained within these domains of the frailty index can be seen as a limitation to the drawing of conclusions beyond the factors that might broadly increase risk. The vigorous debate over this point is further motivating and welcoming inquiries into how we understand the nature of frailty [32].

References

1 Vaupel JW, Manton KG, Stallard E: The impact of heterogeneity in individual frailty on the dynamics of mortality. Demography 1979;16:439–454.

2 Sternberg SA, Wershof Schwartz A, Karunananthan S, et al: The identification of frailty: a systematic literature review. J Am Geriatr Soc 2011;59:2129–2138.

3 Pijpers E, Ferreiraa I, Stehouwera C, et al: The frailty dilemma: review of the predictive accuracy of major frailty scores. Eur J Intern Med 2012;23:118–123.

4 Mitnitski A, Song X, Rockwood K: Assessing biological aging: the origin of deficit accumulation. Biogerontology 2013;14:709–717.

5 Little JDC: Little's law as viewed on its 50th anniversary. Operations Research 2011;59:536–549.

6 Mitnitski A, Song X, Rockwood K: Trajectories of changes over twelve years in the health status of Canadians from late middle age. Exp Gerontol 2012; 47:893–899.

7 Mitnitski A, Mogilner A, Rockwood K: Accumulation of deficits as a proxy measure of aging. ScientificWorldJournal 2001;1:323–336.

8 Rockwood K, Mitnitski A: Frailty defined by deficit accumulation and geriatric medicine defined by frailty. Clin Geriatr Med 2011;27:17–26.

9 Kulminski A, Yashin A, Ukrainsteva S, et al: Accumulation of health disorders as a systemic measure of aging: findings from the NLTCS data. Mech Ageing Dev 2006;127:840–848.

10 Theou O, Brothers TD, Pena F, et al: Identifying common characteristics of frailty across seven scales. J Am Geriatr Soc 2014;62:901–906.

11 Mitnitski A, Song X, Skoog I, et al: Relative fitness and frailty of elderly men and women in developed countries and their relationship with mortality. J Am Geriatr Soc 2005;53:2184–2189.

12 Fried LP, Walston J: Frailty and failure to thrive; in Hazzard W (ed): Principles of Geriatric Medicine and Gerontology. New York, McGraw-Hill, 1998, pp 1387–1402.

13 Fried LP, Tangen C, Walston J, et al: Frailty in older adults: evidence for a phenotype. J Gerontol A Biol Sci Med Sci 2001;56:M146–M156.

14 Chin APM, Dekker JM, Feskens EJ, et al: How to select a frail elderly population? A comparison of three working definitions. J Clin Epidemiol 1999;52:1015–1021.
15 Bandeen-Roche K, Xue Q, Ferrucci L, et al: Phenotype of frailty: characterization in the women's health and aging studies. J Gerontol A Biol Sci Med Sci 2006;61:262–266.
16 Avila-Funes JA, Amieva H, Barberger-Gateau P, et al: Cognitive impairment improves the predictive validity of the phenotype of frailty for adverse health outcomes: the three-city study. J Am Geriatr Soc 2009;57:453–461.
17 Kiely DK, Cupples LA, Lipsitz LA: Validation and comparison of two frailty indexes: the MOBILIZE Boston Study. J Am Geriatr Soc 2009;57:1532–1539.
18 Romero-Ortuno R, Walsh CD, Lawlor BA, et al: A frailty instrument for primary care: findings from the Survey of Health, Ageing and Retirement in Europe (SHARE). BMC Geriatr 2010;10:57.
19 Ensrud KE, Ewing SK, Taylor BC, et al: Comparison of 2 frailty indexes for prediction of falls, disability, fractures, and death in older women. Arch Intern Med 2008;168:382–389.
20 Walston J, McBurnie MA, Newman A, et al: Frailty and activation of the inflammation and coagulation systems with and without clinical morbidities: Results from the Cardiovascular Health Study. Arch Intern Med 2002;162:2333–2341.
21 Leng S, Chaves P, Koenig K, et al: Serum interleukin-6 and hemoglobin as physiological correlates in the geriatric syndrome of frailty: a pilot study. J Am Geriatr Soc 2002;50:1268–1271.
22 Leng S, Yang H, Walston J: Decreased cell proliferation and altered cytokine production in frail older adults. Aging Clin Exp Res 2004;16:249–252.
23 Kalyani RR, Varadhan R, Weiss CO, et al: Frailty status and altered glucose-insulin dynamics. J Gerontol A Biol Sci Med Sci 2012;67:1300–1306.
24 Rolfson DB, Majumdar SR, Tsuyuki RT, et al: Validity and reliability of the Edmonton Frail Scale. Age Ageing 2006;35:526–529.
25 Schuurmans H, Steverink N, Lindenberg S, et al: Old or frail: what tells us more? J Gerontol A Biol Sci Med Sci 2004;59A:M962–M965.
26 Gobbens RJJ, van Assen MALM, Luijkx KG, et al: The Tilburg frailty indicator: psychometric properties. J Am Med Dir Assoc 2010;11:344–355.
27 Abellan VKG, Rolland Y, Bergman H, et al: The I.A.N.A. task force on frailty assessment of older people in clinical practice. J Nutr Health Aging 2008; 12:29–37.
28 Bouillon K, Kivimaki M, Hamer M, et al: Measures of frailty in population-based studies: an overview. BMC Geriatr 2013;13:64.
29 2012 GSA Annual Scientific Meeting Abstracts. The Gerontologist 2012;52(S1):NP.
30 Theou O, Brothers TD, Mitnitski A, et al: Operationalization of frailty using eight commonly used scales and comparison of their ability to predict all-cause mortality. J Am Geriatr Soc 2013;61:1537–1551.
31 Ravindrarajah R, Lee DM, Pye SR, et al: The ability of three different models of frailty to predict all-cause mortality: results from the European Male Aging Study (EMAS). Arch Gerontol Geriatr 2013;57: 360–368.
32 Rodríguez-Mañas L, Féart C, Mann G, et al: Searching for an operational definition of frailty: a Delphi method based consensus statement: the frailty operative definition-consensus conference project. J Gerontol A Biol Sci Med Sci 2013;68:62–67.

Jeremy Walston
Johns Hopkins Asthma and Allergy Center
5501 Hopkins Bayview Circle, Room 1A.62
Baltimore, MD 21224 (USA)
E-Mail jwalston@jhmi.edu

Theou O, Rockwood K (eds): Frailty in Aging. Biological, Clinical and Social Implications.
Interdiscipl Top Gerontol Geriatr. Basel, Karger, 2015, vol 41, pp 74–84 (DOI: 10.1159/000381166)

Comparison and Clinical Applications of the Frailty Phenotype and Frailty Index Approaches

Olga Theou • Kenneth Rockwood

Geriatric Medicine, Faculty of Medicine, Dalhousie University, Halifax, N.S., Canada

Abstract

The previous chapter focused on the conceptualization and operationalization of the deficit accumulation and phenotypic approaches to the description of frailty. The purpose of this chapter is to summarize some studies that compared these most commonly used frailty definitions. We also discuss the strengths and limitations of using these two frailty assessments in clinical settings and how they might be usefully employed in future studies.

The phenotypic and deficit accumulation approaches to the description of frailty agree that frailty is an age-related state of vulnerability to adverse outcomes and that this state arises from a complex interaction of multiple domains, which results in cumulative multisystemic deterioration. While the understanding of frailty has increased exponentially within the past decade, the idea of multisystemic decline is ancient. Hippocrates held that diseases arise from the imbalance of body components ('humors') and that these imbalances produce different diseases with various symptoms. The frailty phenotype and the frailty index also appear to agree that frailty arises when the ability to repair damage falls below the degree of damage originating from the environment or within the organism.

Recent commentators have noted that difficulties in accepting one measure of frailty over another may be due to the ongoing debate over the definition of frailty; as such, it is difficult to create a composite measure that meets all proposed criteria. However, each commonly used frailty scale exhibits shared characteristics: right-

This chapter is based on our previously published work 'Points de repère sur les deux principaux modèles de fragilité: syndrome ou risque, phénotype ou index de fragilité?' in Béland F, Michel H (eds) La fragilité des personnes âgées – Définitions, controverses et perspectives d'action, Rennes, France, Pressses de l'EHESP, 2013, Chapter 1.

skewed density distribution in community-dwelling samples, i.e. most people do not have frailty, but very few people have a large number of deficits; frailty scores that nonlinearly increase with age; mortality risks that increase with increasing frailty scores; higher scores in women than in men, but better survival in women for any degree of frailty; and a maximal upper limit that is below the theoretical maximal score on the scale [1]. Each of these properties is seen in all of the most commonly used frailty measures, with the exception that the frailty phenotype does not show a submaximal limit; i.e. it has a ceiling effect [1].

Comparison of the Nature of the Items Included in the Frailty Index and the Frailty Phenotype

A main area of disagreement between these two operational definitions is the nature of the included items. The group that developed the frailty phenotype [2] proposed that only five domains should be included in the definition of frailty and that this measure should not be applied to parkinsonism or cancer patients, who might meet these criteria on other grounds. A motivation to enable better data collection for fewer items led to the proposal of a simple frailty phenotype that included only three of these domains (weight loss, fatigue, and muscle strength); on the basis of its similar predictive ability for falls, disability, fracture, and mortality compared with the five-item frailty phenotype [3], this method was held to be equivalently useful. In addition, adding cognition as a criterion improved the prediction of adverse health outcomes in a large sample of community-dwelling French older adults [4]; other studies have shown similar results. Disentangling the semantics of the phenotypic definition of frailty is also revealing. The five items that make up the frailty phenotype have been operationalized in different ways by investigators including the originators of this tool [5–7]. This variability limits the comparability of the studies that used the phenotypic operational definition of frailty. A recent study showed that varying the cut-off values of the frailty phenotype from the Cardiovascular Health Study increased the prevalence of frailty from 6.5% to 8.9% in German older adults [8]. Another study of assisted living residents showed that using standard cut-off values resulted in a 19.2% prevalence of frailty but that using the original Cardiovascular Health Study cut-off values resulted in a 48% prevalence of frailty [9].

The frailty index is based on the proposition that knowing what exactly is wrong is less important than knowing how many things are wrong with a person in terms of system behavior. This is the case because the redundancy of complex biological systems results in many ways of achieving the same answer – for example, in the comparability of a dementia diagnosis between psychiatrists, neurologists and geriatricians despite their differences in operationalizing the dementia criteria. For this reason, items should not be excluded a priori, as long as these items meet the criteria described in the previous chapter. It also appears that when more items are included in a frailty index, the specific nature of those deficits is less important in predicting death. For example, 1,000 iterations of 51-item and 40-item frailty indices comprised of different groups of items showed similar dose-response relationships to the risk for mortality and institutionalization [10]. In a separate study, 1,000 iterations of different 37-item frailty indices comprised of different groups of items demonstrated similar hazard ratios for 5-year mortality [11]. In both cases, the level of risk was consistent with the frailty score regardless of the specific nature of the items included in the frailty index, as long as they were generally age-associated and they measured deficits in health. Regardless of the nature and the number of deficits included in the frailty index and whether the sample includes community-dwelling, institutionalized, or hospitalized older adults, the frailty index has remarkably similar measurement properties and substantive results: it shows an age-specific nonlinear increase, women have higher frailty scores than men at any age, it has a maximal limit, and it is strongly associated with adverse health outcomes [12]. Understanding the physical basis for this consistency is an area of intense inquiry.

One persisting conceptual confusion about which items to include reflects the insistence by researchers including the European, Canadian and American Geriatric Advisory Panel that disability and co-morbidity should not be included as part of the definition of frailty since these concepts are conceptually distinct and are a consequence of frailty. This assertion exists as the semantic level, with little empirical evidence to support it, especially in relation to the claim that these aspects are a consequence of the frailty phenotype. This confusion is evident even in the definition of the frailty phenotype, which far from excluding disability, counts impairment in high-order instrumental activities of daily living (gardening, heavy housework) as part of the physical activity criterion. Our group excluded disability and co-morbidity from a frailty index operationalized in the Canadian Study of Health and Aging. Notably, only 3.6% of participants who met the frailty phenotype criteria had neither disability nor co-morbidity, so the distinction appears to largely be without a difference. In any case, for every 0.1 increase in the frailty index score, there was a 21% increase in the 5-year mortality risk when disability and co-morbidity were excluded from the frailty index and a 25–31% increase when they were included [11].

Comparison of the Properties of the Frailty Index and the Frailty Phenotype

Some studies have compared these two approaches to identify which might be more suitable for frailty assessment. A systematic review of frailty assessment tools concluded that the frailty index seems to be the more suitable instrument to evaluate outcome measures in frailty research [13]. They showed that the frailty index includes more items from various domains than the frailty phenotype, and in this way, better covers the multidimensionality of frailty. Even so, in relation to their clinimetric properties, both have only been evaluated for construct validity, mostly because they have been developed as risk assessment tools, not as outcome measures.

Another comparison was made regarding their scoring systems and showed that by having a continuous scoring system, the frailty index can better discriminate and measure change after an intervention [13]. As 'The Frailty Operative Definition-Consensus Conference Project' suggested, 'Frailty is a dynamic nonlinear process', and 'The predictive value of frailty depends of its severity'. Investigators seem to agree on the importance of identifying multiple levels of frailty for both research and clinical purposes. Frailty scores can be dichotomized; however, important information can be lost. For this reason, it is even more important to consider frailty as a continuous score in clinical settings. Similarly to how someone can be hypertensive with a systolic blood pressure of 160 or 180, this person can be frail with a frailty index score of 0.4 or 0.6. Knowing the actual score is at least as important as knowing whether the person is considered to be frail or not.

Many studies have examined the predictive ability of these measures and showed that both the phenotypic operational definition and the frailty index approach have strong predictive validity in relation to worsening health status, poor mobility, activities of daily living disability, institutionalization, and death [2, 12]. Mitnitski et al. [14] compared the ability of the frailty index and the frailty phenotype to predict changes in cognition and mortality using data from the Canadian Study on Health and Aging and showed that both instruments were equally predictive of cognitive decline but that the frailty index was a stronger predictor of mortality. Working from the same dataset, Rockwood and Mitnitski [12] had shown that the two frailty assessments were moderately correlated (r = 0.65) but that the frailty index could predict mortality more precisely. Similarly, Kulminski et al. [15] reported that in the Cardiovascular Health Study (from which the phenotypic definition of frailty was derived), the frailty index more precisely evaluated mortality risk than the frailty phenotype. They found that the frailty phenotype underestimated the risk of death for 720 people, whereas the frailty index underestimated the mortality risk for 134 people. It is important to recall here that mortality risk is not the point of frailty assessment – mortality is convenient to evaluate as a dichotomous, easily verifiable and reasonably non-arbitrary adverse outcome in older adults. Nevertheless, these tools would be expected to underestimate the mortality risk of fitter people who are risk takers, people with genetic profiles that might predispose them to sudden death without substantial deficit accumulation, or those otherwise prone to lethal single-system illness, such as pancreatic cancer.

In older adults residing in assisted living facilities who participated in the Alberta Continuing Care Epidemiological Studies [16], both measures were able to predict mortality, hospitalization, and movement to a long-term care facility for frail people, but only the frailty index predicted these adverse outcomes for people characterized by the phenotypic approach as 'prefrail'. In addition, although both frailty assessments had similar areas under the receiver operating characteristic curve (a measure of sensitivity and specificity) for mortality and hospitalization, the frailty index significantly better discriminated people who moved to a long-term care facility (0.67 vs. 0.61 for the frailty index vs. the frailty phenotype). In a Chinese cohort study of community-dwelling older adults [17], both frailty measures similarly predicted mortality in men and women and physical limitations in men, but the frailty index better discriminated physical limitations in women (AUC 0.66 vs. 0.60). In a European study of community-dwelling people 50+ years of age, the AUC for 2- and 5-year mortality were 0.77 and 0.75, respectively, for the frailty index and 0.73 and 0.70, respectively, for the frailty phenotype. In addition, for participants scoring 0 on the frailty phenotype, the frailty index was able to discriminate participants at a higher risk of death [18].

The frailty index is not meant to be dichotomized into 'frail' or 'healthy' subgroups; even so, for rough classification purposes, a score of 0.25 could generally be considered as a frailty index cut-off score [12]. A recent systematic review [19] that compared the prevalence of frailty in community-dwelling older adults using various assessment tools showed that the weighted average prevalence of frailty was 9.9% using the frailty phenotype; alternatively, in the only included study which used the frailty index, the prevalence of frailty was 22.7%. In older adults residing in assisted living facilities, the prevalence of frailty was 29% when the frailty index approach was used with a cut-off value of 0.3 and was 47.9% when the frailty phenotype was used. Only 38.2% of the participants were assigned to the same categories using both scales (non-frail, prefrail, and frail; kappa = 0.17) [16]. Using data from the Health and Retirement Study, Cigolle et al. [20] found that 11% of older adults were identified as frail based on the frailty phenotype approach and that 32% were identified as frail based on the frailty index approach. In a subsample of this study cohort selected using the same inclusion criteria as the Cardiovascular Health Study, 10.9% were frail based on the frailty phenotype, 15.4% were frail based on the frailty index, and 6.1% were frail based on both measures. Their conclusion was that these frailty assessments capture different subpopulations. Using data from the Survey of Health, Ageing and Retirement in Europe (SHARE), a recent study found that 11% of people over the age of 50 years were identified as frail based on the frailty phenotype approach and that 21% were identified as frail based on the frailty index approach; the level of agreement was 0.51 [18]. In this regard, it is important to note that we cannot say that one measure or the other captures people earlier or later in their health course, as might be expected, for example, if it were simply a matter of sensitivity or specificity. This study also found varying rates of missing data, as have other European studies of community-dwelling older adults, in which people who could not be assessed using the frailty phenotype had higher mortality rates than those who could be assessed [21].

Frailty Assessment in Clinical Settings

The rapid aging of very heterogeneous populations of older adults should be of particular importance to health care providers; for most specialties, the treatment of older adults is the mainstay of their activities. Treating older adults based on risk assessments derived from their chronological age is obviously inappropriate – the rationale for evaluating frailty exists to understand the differential vulnerability of people of the same age to adverse outcomes. For this reason, assessing their level of frailty seems to be a better approach. Frailty is clearly age-related but is distinct from chronological age. A 60-year-old individual who has been identified as very frail may be prescribed high doses of medications and/or undergo medical treatments such as invasive procedures or toxic chemotherapies based on clinical guidelines that have high age-specific limits and may not survive. Factors beyond age explain much of the increased mortality associated with age. Frailty is more strongly associated with worsening of health status, physical function, and self-management skills than chronological age and is also a better predictor of survival and recovery from surgical operations [5, 22–24]. In this way, frailty assessment is a potentially attractive means of understanding risk. We need to consider that not all older adults are frail but that many are, particularly those of older age and those seen in clinical settings. All the above evidence has led clinicians to call frailty the holy grail of geriatric medicine and another geriatric giant.

Frail individuals can be thought of as complex systems that are close to failure and that are vulnerable to further physiological and psychological stressors caused by both intrinsic and environmental factors [12]. Adding one more stressor to such a system, even a stress as minor as one more drug, may lead to death. Considering frail older adults as complex systems close to failure has other advantages, including understanding why illness often presents differently in frail older adults than it does in individuals with a single problem. For example, myocardial ischemia can present without chest pain but with confusion or falls. So-called 'atypical' disease presentations can in fact be typical for frail older adults because when complex systems fail, their highest-order function tends to fail first. This explains the tendency of frail older adults to fall, experience disability and delirium, and become immobile and socially isolated when they are close to failure. In this way, assessing their level of frailty is a more important determinant of health status than an individual pathophysiological pathway.

Frailty can assist clinicians in identifying patients who might benefit more from innovative processes of care than from aggressive medical treatments and can improve the health outcomes of individuals across various clinical settings. Clinicians can use the information from frailty assessments to discuss with patients and caregivers the risks and benefits of possible treatments, which can lead to a more informed and rational shared decision. Frailty assessment could start from primary care since family physicians focus more on patient-centered care and are able to take into consideration the social context of the patients and how their social context affects their health status. A frailty index constructed using administrative routine health care data from general practitioners showed that increasing the frailty index score by one deficit increases the hazard of adverse health outcomes by 17% [25]. Even so, in that study, frailty was operationalized chiefly in relation to comorbidity, perhaps reflecting a legacy of a primary care focus on episodic treatment of acute illness that has been hard to shake, even as an emphasis on chronic disease management has grown.

Operationalizing frailty in primary care seems both feasible and valuable. For example, an analysis of data from the Medicare Current Beneficiary Survey showed that frailty increases the risk of adverse outcomes after emergency department discharge by 45% [26]. Frailty also predicts the toxicity of chemotherapy in older patients with cancer [27]. In a study including patients undergoing colorectal cancer resection, the odds ratio of major postoperative complications was 4.08 for frail patients [28]. In colectomy patients, the frailty index was an important predictor of intensive care unit complications and death [29]. In addition, there is a paucity of data on the strong relationship between frailty and cardiovascular disease outcomes. A systematic review of patients with cardiovascular disease showed that the presence of frailty increased the risk of mortality; mortality at 9 years was 100% when the level of frailty was high and was 55% when the level of frailty was low [30]. Frailty has also been found to be an important risk factor for dementia.

For these reasons, frailty seems a reasonable candidate for assessment in clinical settings. Even so, many clinicians remain unpersuaded about the feasibility of frailty assessments in routine care and believe that clinical judgment should not be replaced by objective frailty measures. Different clinicians have different perceptions of frailty, which can result in different kinds of people being identified as frail. This discrepancy emphasizes the importance of using standardized, objective measures of frailty across disciplines. The frailty phenotype approach has widely been used in research due to the easy measurability of its 5 components, but it seems to be impractical in clinical settings, especially due to the inclusion of performance-based measures, which many older adults are too impaired to complete safely. One study operationalizing frailty based on this approach in residents of assisted living facilities found that 40% of the residents were unable to be assessed [9].

One important point in comparing the frailty index with the frailty phenotype is that frailty itself is clearly not all or none – degrees of frailty are clinically evident and empirically demonstrable – but the three-level operational definition of frailty seems to overlook this aspect. For example, the frailty phenotype was not predictive of health care use such as emergency department visits [31] and only marginally improved the prediction of select adverse outcomes for assisted living residents [9].

That the frailty index approach can be developed from any existing biomedical database is a strength: not every frailty index need include the same items. As it can be constructed by using self-reported measures, it is feasible even for individuals who are unable to undertake performance-based tests. An important drawback is that it requires that at least 20 items be considered, which has made clinicians skeptical about its feasibility. Although many more than 20 items are included in a comprehensive geriatric assessment, this number of items is more than the number of items that is normally considered for screening. In addition, though the frailty index is well validated and investigated in clinical settings, some have asserted that the frailty index is more useful for policy planners than for clinicians [32]. The basis for this assertion is unclear, especially in the era of electronic health records, in which a large number of items is routinely available for consideration. Even though the operationalization of both the frailty phenotype and the frailty index has limitations, assessing frailty is important for clinical care, research, and policy planning, and there is little doubt about its impact on older individuals, families and society as a whole.

Frailty Screening

Frailty screening can identify 'at risk' patients who will benefit from a comprehensive assessment in which clinicians can make a precise diagnosis of frailty and examine in more depth the multiple and interacting problems that affect the health status of their patients [33]. An effective frailty screening tool should follow the World Health Organization guidelines regarding population screening: (a) commonness and importance to public health, (b) the availability of specific and sensitive tests for detection, (c) recognizable early stages, (d) the availability of effective treatments, and (e) a more beneficial than harmful screening process.

Most researchers and clinicians would agree on the importance of frailty assessment in clinical settings. However, there is no agreement on frailty screening. Some believe that screening for frailty should be an essential part of the care of older adults, especially those facing medical treatment decisions [32], whereas others are less persuaded about the likelihood of its success [34]. The former group emphasizes the strong predictive validity of frailty screening for identifying people at high risk of adverse events and the potential of frailty screening to lead to the more targeted assessment of people who need them and to end the unnecessary assessment of severely frail people. The latter group emphasizes that there is not enough evidence about the sensitivity of the frailty scales in order to use them as screening tools and that there may be other adverse events associated with the screening such as labelling people as frail and adding one more item to the long and burdensome list of screenings that older adults have to go through [34].

There is no clear agreement on a frailty screening tool that is appropriate for both clinicians and epidemiologists. The frailty phenotype and frailty index approaches are not simple enough, and they include more items that what is normally included in screening. A possible candidate screening measure could be the Clinical Frailty Scale [35]. The Clinical Frailty Scale is based on the clinical evaluation of a patient's status in the domains of mobility, energy, physical activity, and function and is now expanded to include nine levels: very fit, well, managing well, vulnerable, mildly frail, moderately frail, severely frail, very severely frail, and terminally ill. In addition, gait speed could represent a suitable screening tool, as its assessment is quick and inexpensive and it is proven to be a highly reliable measure of adverse outcomes. Even though both frailty screening and assessment seem important for the care of older adults, how these would be incorporated into everyday care in clinical settings and how they would benefit clinical decisions need to be foci of translational research programs.

Future Studies

As understanding frailty continues to motivate research by geriatricians, laboratory-based scientists, epidemiologists, and sociologists, studies should further examine the usage of the frailty phenotype and frailty index approaches in clinical care, research, and policy planning and should reach an agreement for a standardized frailty assessment tool across settings or for which tool should be used in each setting. Another approach could be to use both assessment tools when frailty is examined. In addition, more studies are needed regarding the ability of these measures to be used as frailty screening tools and as outcome measures for intervention studies and the role of biological markers in their operationalization. Another potential future area of investigation is the ability to incorporate medical information systems to screen and assess frailty. Knowledge translation studies should focus on how the frailty phenotype and the frailty index should be used across settings. Education on the importance of assessing frailty for decision making and on the appropriate usage of the assessment results should be provided to health care professionals, especially those who regularly treat reasonably independent, community-dwelling older adults.

References

1 Theou O, Brothers TD, Pena F, Mitnitski A, Rockwood K: Identifying common characteristics of frailty across seven scales. J Am Geriatr Soc 2014;62:901–906.

2 Fried LP, Tangen CM, Walston J, Newman AB, Hirsch C, Gottdiener J, Seeman T, Tracy R, Kop WJ, Burke G, McBurnie MA; Cardiovascular Health Study Collaborative Research Group: Frailty in older adults: evidence for a phenotype. J Gerontol A Biol Sci Med Sci 2001;56:M146–M156.

3 Ensrud KE, Ewing SK, Cawthon PM, Fink HA, Taylor BC, Cauley JA, Dam TT, Marshall LM, Orwoll ES, Cummings SR; Osteoporotic Fractures in Men Research Group: A comparison of frailty indexes for the prediction of falls, disability, fractures, and mortality in older men. J Am Geriatr Soc 2009;57:492–498.

4 Avila-Funes JA, Amieva H, Barberger-Gateau P, Le Goff M, Raoux N, Ritchie K, Carrière I, Tavernier B, Tzourio C, Gutiérrez-Robledo LM, Dartigues JF: Cognitive impairment improves the predictive validity of the phenotype of frailty for adverse health outcomes: the three-city study. J Am Geriatr Soc 2009;57:453–461.

5 Makary MA, Segev DL, Pronovost PJ, Syin D, Bandeen-Roche K, Patel P, Takenaga R, Devgan L, Holzmueller CG, Tian J, Fried LP: Frailty as a predictor of surgical outcomes in older patients. J Am Coll Surg 2010;210:901–908.

6 Varadhan R, Walston J, Cappola AR, Carlson MC, Wand GS, Fried LP: Higher levels and blunted diurnal variation of cortisol in frail older women. J Gerontol A Biol Sci Med Sci 2008;63:190–195.

7 Bartali B, Frongillo EA, Bandinelli S, Lauretani F, Semba RD, Fried LP, Ferrucci L: Low nutrient intake is an essential component of frailty in older persons. J Gerontol A Biol Sci Med Sci 2006;61:589–593.
8 Saum KU, Müller H, Stegmaier C, Hauer K, Raum E, Brenner H: Development and evaluation of a modification of the Fried frailty criteria using population-independent cutpoints. J Am Geriatr Soc 2012;60: 2110–2115.
9 Freiheit EA, Hogan DB, Strain LA, Schmaltz HN, Patten SB, Eliasziw M, Maxwell CJ: Operationalizing frailty among older residents of assisted living facilities. BMC Geriatr 2011;11:23.
10 Rockwood K, Mitnitski A, Song X, Steen B, Skoog I: Long-term risks of death and institutionalization of elderly people in relation to deficit accumulation at age 70. J Am Geriatr Soc 2006;54:975–979.
11 Theou O, Rockwood MR, Mitnitski A, Rockwood K: Disability and co-morbidity in relation to frailty: how much do they overlap? Arch Gerontol Geriatr 2012;55:e1–e8.
12 Rockwood K, Mitnitski A: Frailty defined by deficit accumulation and geriatric medicine defined by frailty. Clin Geriatr Med 2011;27:17–26.
13 de Vries NM, Staal JB, van Ravensberg CD, Hobbelen JS, Olde Rikkert MG, Nijhuis-van der Sanden MW: Outcome instruments to measure frailty: a systematic review. Ageing Res Rev 2011;10:104–114.
14 Mitnitski A, Fallah N, Rockwood MR, Rockwood K: Transitions in cognitive status in relation to frailty in older adults: a comparison of three frailty measures. J Nutr Health Aging 2011;15:863–867.
15 Kulminski AM, Ukraintseva SV, Kulminskaya IV, Arbeev KG, Land K, Yashin AI: Cumulative deficits better characterize susceptibility to death in elderly people than phenotypic frailty: lessons from the Cardiovascular Health Study. J Am Geriatr Soc 2008;56: 898–903.
16 Hogan DB, Freiheit EA, Strain LA, Patten SB, Schmaltz HN, Rolfson D, Maxwell CJ: Comparing frailty measures in their ability to predict adverse outcome among older residents of assisted living. BMC Geriatr 2012;12:56.
17 Woo J, Leung J, Morley JE: Comparison of frailty indicators based on clinical phenotype and the multiple deficit approach in predicting mortality and physical limitation. J Am Geriatr Soc 2012;60:1478–1486.
18 Theou O, Brothers TD, Mitnitski A, Rockwood K: Operationalization of frailty using eight commonly used scales and comparison of their ability to predict all-cause mortality. J Am Geriatr Soc 2013;61:1537–1551.
19 Collard RM, Boter H, Schoevers RA, Oude Voshaar RC: Prevalence of frailty in community-dwelling older persons: a systematic review. J Am Geriatr Soc 2012;60:1487–1492.
20 Cigolle CT, Ofstedal MB, Tian Z, Blaum CS: Comparing models of frailty: the Health and Retirement Study. J Am Geriatr Soc 2009;57:830–839.
21 Ravindrarajah R, Lee DM, Pye SR, Gielen E, Boonen S, Vanderschueren D, Pendleton N, Finn JD, Tajar A, O'Connell MD, Rockwood K, Bartfai G, Casanueva FF, Forti G, Giwercman A, Han TS, Huhtaniemi IT, Kula K, Lean ME, Punab M, Wu FC, O'Neill TW; European Male Aging Study Group: The ability of three different models of frailty to predict all-cause mortality: results from the European Male Aging Study (EMAS). Arch Gerontol Geriatr 2013;57:360–368.
22 Robinson TN, Eiseman B, Wallace JI: Redefining geriatric preoperative assessment using frailty, disability and co-morbidity. Ann Surg 2009;250:449–455.
23 Brown NA, Zenilman ME: The impact of frailty in the elderly on the outcome of surgery in the aged. Adv Surg 2010;44:229–249.
24 Theou O, Jones G, Jakobi J, Mitnitski A, Vandervoort A: A comparison of the relationship of 14 performance-based measures with frailty in older women. Appl Physiol Nutr Metab 2011;36:928–938.
25 Drubbel I, de Wit NJ, Bleijenberg N, Eijkemans RJ, Schuurmans MJ, Numans ME: Prediction of adverse health outcomes in older people using a frailty index based on routine primary care data. J Gerontol A Biol Sci Med Sci 2013;68:301–308.
26 Hastings SN, Purser JL, Johnson KS, Sloane RJ, Whitson HE: Frailty predicts some but not all adverse outcomes in older adults discharged from the emergency department. J Am Geriatr Soc 2008;56: 1651–1657.
27 Hamaker ME, Vos AG, Smorenburg CH, de Rooij SE, van Munster BC: The value of geriatric assessments in predicting treatment tolerance and all-cause mortality in older patients with cancer. Oncologist 2012;17:1439–1449.
28 Tan KY, Kawamura YJ, Tokomitsu A, Tang T: Assessment for frailty is useful for predicting morbidity in elderly patients undergoing colorectal cancer resection whose comorbidities are already optimized. Am J Surg 2012;204:139–143.
29 Obeid NM, Azuh O, Reddy S, Webb S, Reickert C, Velanovich V, Horst HM, Rubinfeld I: Predictors of critical care-related complications in colectomy patients using the National Surgical Quality Improvement Program: exploring frailty and aggressive laparoscopic approaches. J Trauma Acute Care Surg 2012;72:878–883.
30 Afilalo J, Karunananthan S, Eisenberg MJ, Alexander KP, Bergman H: Role of frailty in patients with cardiovascular disease. Am J Cardiol 2009;103: 1616–1621.

31 Au A, Puts MT, Fletcher JD, Sourial N, Bergman H: Frailty markers predicting emergency department visits in a community-dwelling sample of vulnerable seniors in Montreal. Can J Aging 2011;30:647–655.
32 Sternberg SA, Wershof Schwartz A, Karunananthan S, Bergman H, Mark Clarfield A: The identification of frailty: a systematic literature review. J Am Geriatr Soc 2011;59:2129–2138.
33 Theou O, Rockwood K: Should frailty status always be considered when treating the elderly patient? Aging Health 2012;8:261–271.
34 Pijpers E, Ferreiraa I, Stehouwera C, Nieuwenhuijzen Krusemana A: The frailty dilemma: review of the predictive accuracy of major frailty scores. Eur J Intern Med 2012;23:118–123.
35 Morley JE, Vellas B, van Kan GA, Anker SD, Bauer JM, Bernabei R, Cesari M, Chumlea WC, Doehner W, Evans J, Fried LP, Guralnik JM, Katz PR, Malmstrom TK, McCarter RJ, Gutierrez Robledo LM, Rockwood K, von Haehling S, Vandewoude MF, Walston J: Frailty consensus: a call to action. J Am Med Dir Assoc 2013;14:392–397.

Dr. Olga Theou
5955 Veterans' Memorial Lane
Suite 1313
Halifax, NS B3H 2E1 (Canada)
E-Mail otheou@alumni.uwo.ca

Theou O, Rockwood K (eds): Frailty in Aging. Biological, Clinical and Social Implications.
Interdiscipl Top Gerontol Geriatr. Basel, Karger, 2015, vol 41, pp 85–94 (DOI: 10.1159/000381170)

Frailty in Primary Care

Roman Romero-Ortuno

Department of Medicine for the Elderly, Addenbrooke's Hospital, Cambridge University Hospitals NHS Foundation Trust, Cambridge, UK

Abstract

This chapter considers the pragmatic integration of frailty in primary care. While some patients present to primary care practitioners with relatively well-defined problems that can be managed by a single intervention and/or organ-specific specialist referral, others present with nonacute, poorly defined problems that are *complex* and rooted in multiple factors. The latter are often in need of a comprehensive geriatric assessment (CGA). CGA can have important positive impacts on the health of older people, but it is labor-intensive and costly. Therefore, patients at *higher risk* of adverse outcomes should have *higher priority* to publicly funded CGA services. Frailty is an age-independent *marker of risk* that fits the biopsychosocial model of primary care, and its use (as opposed to age alone) may promote *equity of access* to CGA services. A number of frailty assessment tools have been recommended for use in primary care. Some randomized controlled trials have shown that frailty screening in primary care, with subsequent CGA and intervention, can prevent adverse outcomes. However, this result has not been obtained with every screening tool, and comparative trials are ongoing. Meanwhile, primary care commissioners in the UK are establishing new frailty care pathways and developing *frailty registers* in primary care.

Around the world, populations are aging. In Europe, by 2060, those aged 65+ will comprise 30% of the population, and one person in eight will be aged 80 years or more. Even so, it is well recognized that the association between age and health status is extremely variable in the older population [1]. On the one hand, the majority of community-dwelling older people enjoy good physical and cognitive health and often present to primary care practitioners with 'single', relatively well-defined problems that can be managed by a single intervention and/or organ-specific specialist referral.

On the other hand, a minority of older patients present with nonacute, poorly defined problems (e.g. 'tired all the time', recurrent falls, 'failure to thrive', or gradual cognitive and/or functional decline). These patients are complex because their presentation is rooted in multiple factors, including morbidity (e.g. physical or cognitive), polypharmacy, psychosocial influences and social vulnerability, in varying degrees and combinations. In primary care, for which consultation times and access to multidisciplinary assessments are limited, unraveling this complexity for the first time can prove to be challenging. Thus, these more complex patients often need a comprehensive geriatric assessment (CGA).

CGA is defined as a multidisciplinary diagnostic and intervention process that identifies physical, cognitive, environmental, psychosocial and socioeconomic components that influence the health of older adults. CGA is based on the premise that a systematic and personalized evaluation may identify remediable problems and that by tackling them in a coordinated manner, the risk of adverse outcomes for the person will be minimized [2].

CGA can provide important positive impacts on health care for older people, including more thorough diagnoses and improved levels of physical and psychological functioning [3]. However, these benefits have costs. Considering its usual interdisciplinary composition and the time that it takes to gather relevant data, CGA is labor-intensive and not inexpensive. Therefore, from the point of view of both the referrers and providers of CGA, it is important to identify those who need it the most to promote equitable access to this vital (but finite), expert, multidisciplinary resource. Although no explicit criteria have been validated to readily identify patients who are likely to benefit from CGA [2], chronological age alone is unlikely to identify vulnerable patients given the great biological heterogeneity of the population of older people [1]. Rather, it would be fair to say that patients at *higher risk* of adverse outcomes should have *higher priority* to publicly funded CGA services. This approach pursues *equality of access for equal need* as a form of equity in publicly funded health and social care services [4].

Frailty: An Age-Independent Marker of Risk that Fits the Biopsychosocial Model of Primary Care

In primary care, for which consultation times and multidisciplinary resources are limited, the concept of *frailty* may have a very good fit as a *risk stratification paradigm* that is rooted in the biopsychosocial model of primary care. Indeed, frailty is defined (regardless of chronological age) as *vulnerability to adverse outcomes* due to the poor resolution of homoeostasis after stressor events [5]. Conceptually, it has been argued that frailty fits well with the biopsychosocial model of general practice and may provide commissioners of health care with a clinical focus for targeting resources to an aging population [6]. Indeed, 'family physicians are ideally suited to incorporate the concept of frailty into their practice because they have the propensity and skill set that lends itself to patient-centered care, taking into account the individual subtleties of the patient's health within their social context' [7].

For the purpose of individual risk stratification and CGA prioritization, a good frailty tool in primary care should fulfill the following criteria: (1) be a reliable risk marker (i.e. have been shown to predict adverse outcomes); (2) be of multidimensional nature (i.e. include, or be closely related to, key biopsychosocial variables); (3) be easily measurable in primary care (i.e. brief and easy to administer); (4) be breakable into risk categories (i.e. low vs. high risk, with or without an intermediate risk category or categories); and (5) be easily understandable by CGA providers (so that CGA referrals can be adequately and systematically prioritized).

In recent years, considerable progress has been made in determining operational definitions of frailty. While various approaches exist, the commonality among them all is the concept of frailty as a *marker of risk* for adverse outcomes, independent of chronological age [5]. The following sections review the two main approaches to the operationalization of frailty, namely the *frailty index* (FI; i.e. frailty as a state) and the *frailty phenotype* (i.e. frailty as a syndrome), and examine their suitabilities for the risk stratification of nonacute, complex, older patients in primary care.

The Frailty Index in Primary Care

One way to operationalize frailty is by considering it *as a state* and counting the number of *deficits* an individual has accumulated from a given list (of usually 30 or more potential deficits). Deficits are widely defined as symptoms, signs, diseases and disabilities that accumulate with age [8]. The number of counted deficits divided by the number of deficits considered results in a score called the FI, which ranges from 0 (none of the deficits present) to 1 (all deficits present).

The construct validity of the FI is examined through its relationship with chronological age, and its criterion validity is evaluated according to its ability to predict mortality [9] and in relation to other predictions, including disability and the use of health care resources [10]. In a primary care context, an advantage of the FI approach is that it tends to include a wide range of deficits, making the assessment biopsychosocial from the outset. In addition, there is evidence that the FI is associated with social determinants of health, which help to clarify the wide range of 'biological ages' within population subgroups of the same chronological age [10].

In terms of individual risk stratification, the FI is a continuous variable that does not primarily classify people as frail or nonfrail; rather, it assigns a score based on health status. Because the FI score ranges from 0 to 1, it can be easily understood by CGA providers. In addition, Rockwood et al. have proposed FI cut-off points to define population subgroups with increasing levels of frailty. For example, in one of their studies, they have proposed an FI of ≤0.08 as 'non-frail', an FI of ≥0.25 as 'frail', and the remainder of the scores as 'pre-frail' [11]. In another of their studies, they have proposed an FI of ≤0.03 as 'relatively fit', 0.03< FI ≤0.10 as 'less fit', 0.10< FI ≤0.21 as 'least fit', 0.21< FI ≤0.45 as 'frail', and FI ≥0.45 as 'most frail' [12]. Using these FI cut-off points, primary care practitioners can also stratify individual patient risk, which may help CGA providers in terms of the prioritization of referrals.

Another advantage of the FI is that it can be tailored to existing data collection and allows flexibility in the choice of deficits as long as they comply with a simple set of required properties [8]. However, given the number of deficits required (usually 30 or more), an FI may take some time to be determined in primary care. Computer versions of the FI that are integrated into routine electronic data collection during consultation may be suitable for implementing the FI in primary care. An example is an FI based on International Classification of Primary Care (ICPC)-encoded routine health care data, which has been shown to predict the risks of adverse health outcomes in a population of older people attending primary care [13].

The Frailty Phenotype in Primary Care

According to the phenotypic approach, frailty is defined as a clinical syndrome in which three or more of the following criteria are present: *unintentional weight loss*, self-reported *exhaustion*, *weakness*, *slow walking speed*, and *low physical activity* [14]. This approach defines two additional states, pre-frail (i.e. one or two criteria present) and nonfrail (i.e. none of the criteria present), conforming to a three-category ordinal variable. The original validation of this approach by Fried et al. included significant associations with incident disease, hospitalization, falls, disability and mortality [14], making it another suitable risk stratification scheme for the purpose of prioritizing CGA referrals.

An advantage of this approach is that it requires the measurement of only five variables, which makes the frailty assessment relatively quick. While this approach is feasible from a primary care point of view, a problem arises with the construction of the tool. In Fried's definition [14], frailty is defined in terms of three categories, each of which is defined by the sum of the number of individual criteria present (0: *nonfrail*; 1 or 2: *pre-frail*; and 3, 4 or 5: *frail*). The dichotomization of individual criterion that are measured on a continuous scale (i.e. grip strength, walking speed and physical activity) is performed retrospectively according to the lowest twentieth percentile rule, and there are further stratifications. This requires post hoc statistical analyses of a reference sample, which is not always available to primary care practitioners.

Because surrogates for individual frailty phenotype criteria are available [15], there have been attempts to provide primary care practitioners with phenotypic frailty assessment tools that do not require post hoc calculations and can be scored immediately after an individual patient assessment. An example of the latter is the *Frailty Instrument for Primary Care of the Survey of Health, Aging and Retirement in Europe* (SHARE-FI) [16]. This tool is based on a modified phenotypic approach and includes two web-based frailty calculators (one for each gender) that are freely accessible on *BMC Geriatrics* web page (http://www.biomedcentral.com/1471–2318/10/57/additional). Their uses are intended for community-dwelling adults aged 50 and over. Translated versions of the calculators can be accessed on https://sites.google.com/a/tcd.ie/share-frailty-instrument-calculators/. The SHARE-FI has been validated against incident disability [17] and predicts mortality similar to the FI based on CGA [18]. In a recent observational study carried out in a geriatric day care facility, people identified as frail by the SHARE-FI had worse physical performance scores, an increased history of falls, a greater medication burden and were more often referred for ongoing multidisciplinary assessment and rehabilitation [19]. An advantage of the SHARE-FI is that, on average, it only takes about 6.5 minutes to administer (http://www.uakron.edu/dotAsset/8b117eba-ec49-4e57-9495-fe41fcfbd995.pdf).

Frailty Tools in Primary Care: Recommendations from Systematic Reviews

A number of reviews have addressed the suitability of frailty assessment tools for the purpose of risk stratification in primary care. A recent systematic review by Pialoux et al. [20] compared the properties of ten frailty screening tools for primary care, which were selected from the literature according to the following premises: (1) the tools were multidimensional in nature; (2) they had been compared to a more complete geriatric evaluation or to a CGA measurement tool; and (3) they had been tested in a primary health care setting and/or in a nonhospitalized population. The following instruments were considered by Pialoux et al.: (1) a *postal screening questionnaire* by Barber et al.; (2) the *Sherbrooke Postal Questionnaire* (SPQ); (3) the *functional assessment screening package* by Moore and Siu; (4) the *screening instrument* by Maly et al.; (5) the *Strawbridge questionnaire*; (6) the *PRISMA-7* case finding tool; (7) the *Brief Risk Identification of Geriatric Health Tool* (BRIGHT) postal questionnaire; (8) a *self-administered test* based on the Marigliano-Cacciafesta polypathological scale (MCPS); (9) the *Tilburg Frailty Indicator* (TFI); and (10) the SHARE-FI. Pialoux et al. have concluded that it is difficult to determine which tool is the best for screening for frailty in older people in primary care settings but that two instruments were potentially suitable – the TFI and the SHARE-FI. However, it was pointed out that these instruments require validation with larger studies in primary health care settings using more quality criteria [20].

The *Oxford Center for Monitoring and Diagnosis in Primary Care* (MADOX) recently carried out a systematic review of screening instruments for frailty in primary care (Horizon Scan Report 0026, 8 November 2012, http://madox.org/horizon-scanning-reports/20120026/screening-instruments-for-frailty-in-primary-care). In their review, the authors described the following instruments, selected for their relevance to primary care: the *Emergency Admission Risk Likelihood Index* (EARLI), SHARE-FI, SPQ, TFI, the *Identification of Seniors at Risk* (ISAR) tool, the *8-item Runciman* questionnaire, the *7-item Rowland* questionnaire, the *abbreviated comprehensive geriatric assessment* (aCGA) tool, the *G8* tool, the *Groningen Frailty Indicator* (GFI), and the *Vulnerable Elders Survey* (VES-13) tool. The MADOX review concluded that because there is no gold standard to measure frailty and because different instruments have been tested in different settings and with different outcome measures, it is not possible to select one screening tool for the identification of frail older people.

However, it has been concluded that eight of the identified tools may be good screening instruments, including the SHARE-FI and TFI (as also identified by Pialoux et al. [20]), and the GFI, 7-item Rowland, G8, VES-13, ISAR, and aCGA.

Recently, a consensus group consisting of delegates from six major international, European, and US societies provided examples of well-validated frailty models [21], including phenotypic and index approaches. According to this consensus document, well-validated frailty models include recommended screening tools for primary care, such as the SHARE-FI and TFI (as recommended by Pialoux et al. and the MADOX) and the VES-13 and GFI (as also recommended by the MADOX). In addition, other primary care-friendly instruments were highlighted in the consensus document, such as the *FRAIL scale* from the International Academy of Nutrition and Aging, the *Clinical Frailty Scale*, the *Study of Osteoporotic Fractures* (SOF) FI, and the *Gérontopôle Frailty Screening Tool.* This group agreed that all of these instruments can be used to identify persons who are in need of a more in-depth assessment [21].

Importantly, comparative epidemiological studies have shown that many of these tools have similar risk-prediction abilities [9]; therefore, the primary care practitioner should select, among all of the validated and recommended tools, the one that is freely and easily available, suitable for his/her particular primary care environment, and can be administered within the available time frame and with the available resources. In addition, the choice of screening tool may be supported by the results of randomized controlled trials and prior local clinical experience.

Frailty Screening and Intervention in Primary Care: Randomized Controlled Trials

As outlined above, there are many frailty screening tools suitable for primary care, and at present, none can be identified as 'the best'. However, the key question is whether frailty screening in primary care is fulfilling in terms of its remit of improving outcomes for patients in real practice by facilitating preferential access to CGA and interventions. This question has been examined by some randomized controlled trials.

FRAilty, Screening and Intervention (FRASI), a randomized controlled trial aimed at preventing activities of daily living (ADL) disability in frail older persons screened in primary care, used the *Short Physical Performance Battery* (SPPB) to screen for frailty. Frail participants were randomized into treatment and control groups, and the active group received an intensive medical intervention and sixteen 90-minute supervised exercise sessions over a period of 8 weeks. The primary outcome was time to ADL disability onset or death in the 12-month period after study enrollment. The results suggested that screening in primary care of nondisabled, older persons with frailty (i.e. an SPPB of ≤9) can identify individuals with substantial morbidity, impairments and functional limitations who can successfully undergo intensive medical and exercise interventions [22].

However, a recent cluster randomized controlled trial has yielded negative results in this regard [23]. In this trial, frail older people in primary care were selected on the basis of a GFI score of ≥5. Practices in the control group delivered care as usual, and those in the intervention group implemented the 'Prevention of Care' approach, in which frail older people received a multidimensional assessment and interdisciplinary care based on a tailor-made treatment plan and regular evaluations and follow-ups. At 24 months, there were no significant differences between the two groups in terms of disability (primary outcome) or other adverse outcomes [23].

Notwithstanding the abovementioned findings, another randomized controlled trial assessed the effectiveness of CGA and subsequent intervention in pre-frail and frail community-dwelling elderly based on Fried's frailty phenotype criteria and found that CGA and subsequent intervention resulted in a favorable outcome based on frailty status and the Barthel index of ADL [24].

It is possible that the uses of different frailty screening tools in primary care-based trials may influence their outcomes, and the simultaneous comparison of various frailty-screening tools in primary care is an emerging area of research. An example is the ongoing single-blind, three-armed, cluster-randomized controlled trial with a one-year follow-up called the *Utrecht Primary care PROactive Frailty Intervention Trial* (U-PROFIT) [25]. In this trial, 58 general practices in the Netherlands, with approximately 5,000 older individuals, are expected to participate. This ambitious study will compare the following three interventions: (1) the performance of a computerized, primary care-friendly FI assessment based on routine health care data, which will periodically prioritize patients for general practitioner (GP) assessment (this arm is called *U-PRIM*); (2) the use of the GFI to identify frail patients, with a subsequent nurse-led CGA at home and a tailor-made care plan developed by a nurse and GP based on the outcome of the CGA (i.e. *U-CARE* model); and (3) primary care as usual. The primary outcome is the effects on ADL as measured with the Katz ADL index. Secondary outcomes are quality of life, mortality, nursing home admission, emergency department, out-of-hours general practice visits, and caregiver burden.

New Commissioning Models in Primary Care: Examples from the United Kingdom

Although the evidence from randomized trials is (although promising) still not conclusive for the effectiveness of frailty screening in primary care, in countries such as the UK, there is currently a drive for the integration of health and social care at the community level, and many primary care commissioners are establishing new dedicated frailty care pathways and developing *frailty registers* in primary care. While these innovative (and quality improvement-driven) clinical programs are still at early developmental stages, their future evaluations will provide a valuable complement to the evidence emerging from clinical trials.

For example, the *Mid Essex Clinical Commissioning Group* (http://www.midessexccg.nhs.uk/) is developing a frailty register in general practice clinical systems and will create a database of activity and costs (including social care) for identified cohorts of these at-risk individuals. Their intention is to develop a 'year of care' tariff and to commission an 'accountable lead provider' to provide out-of-hospital health (and social) care to frail older people to reduce unplanned hospital admissions.

In London, the *Camden Clinical Commissioning Group* (http://www.camdenccg.nhs.uk/) has designed and implemented an Integrated Patient-Centered Care (IPCC) program for frail adults. In this program, identifying people for integrated patient-centered case management relies on the *Edmonton Frail Scale* (EFS). Any patient scoring 10 or more on the EFS will receive integrated working-enhanced services, involving the appointment of a case manager who will undertake a home-based CGA and work with the GP and community multidisciplinary services to design tailored interventions and provide ongoing patient reviews.

It is likely that financial incentives to primary care practices will increase the popularity of frailty screening in primary care for the purpose of proactive integrated case management in the community. For example, the *Cumbria Clinical Commissioning Group* (http://www.cumbriaccg.nhs.uk/) will incentivize primary care practices by paying them £80 for each completed proactive care plan for patients identified on the frailty register. Following frailty screening, the proactive plan includes a home visit, CGA, intervention/s and subsequent monitoring and reviews (http://www.cumbriaccg.nhs.uk/about-us/how-we-make-decisions/governing-body-meetings/2013/2013–05–09/papers/7-part2-gp-incentive-scheme-paper.pdf).

Summary and Conclusions

On initial 'eyeball' assessment of a nonacute, complex patient, the experienced primary care practitioner will *intuitively* know when a referral for CGA is indicated, and the use of frailty screening tools is unlikely to be a substitute for that expert clinical impression. However, providers of CGA need to prioritize their referrals, and the age-independent risk stratification offered by frailty screening tools can externally validate the eyeball test and increase the transparency and equity of access to CGA services. It is in this regard that family physicians and community practitioners need easy-to-use frailty screening instruments [26].

The measurement of frailty in primary care is ideally suited to the nonacute, undiagnosed, complex older adult who is considered to be vulnerable and in need of CGA. Frailty, as an age-independent risk marker, will help to prioritize those who may benefit from access to CGA; in turn, CGA will help to diagnose the underlying cause/s of frailty and reduce vulnerability. Ensuring that those who are frailer have sooner access to CGA is not only more equitable, but it may also help to reduce the incidence of frailty-related adverse outcomes, such as hospitalizations and institutionalizations. The use of objective frailty metrics in primary care is mainly for adopting a *language of communication* between primary care and CGA providers to enable equity of access to publicly funded CGA resources. In a time of limited resources, frailty has the potential to become an advocacy and policy tool. The results from randomized clinical trials and the experiences of novel clinical programs will clarify whether this potential will become a reality.

Appendix

Examples of Easily Available Frailty Screening Tools for Primary Care

Tilburg Frailty Indicator (TFI): http://www.tilburguniversity.edu/upload/ac3c1079–6188–4bea-b4af-8f552c07a1d2_tfieng.pdf
SHARE Frailty Instrument for primary care (SHARE-FI): http://www.biomedcentral.com/1471–2318/10/57/additional
Groningen Frailty Indicator (GFI): http://www.biomedcentral.com/1471–2318/13/86/additional
Vulnerable Elders Survey (VES-13): http://www.rand.org/health/projects/acove/survey.html
Clinical Frailty Scale (CFS): http://geriatricresearch.medicine.dal.ca/pdf/Clinical%20Faily%20Scale.pdf
The FRAIL questionnaire screening tool (3 or greater = frailty; 1 or 2 = pre-frail): ***F****atigue: Are you fatigued?* ***R****esistance: Can you walk up 1 flight of stairs?* ***A****erobic: Can you walk 1 block?* ***I****llnesses: Do you have more than 5 illnesses?* ***L****oss of weight: Have you lost more than 5% of your weight in the past 6 months?*
Short Physical Performance Battery (SPPB): http://web.missouri.edu/~proste/tool/ShortPhysicalPerformanceBattery.pdf
Edmonton Frail Scale (EFS): https://itunes.apple.com/us/app/edmonton-frail-scale-for-ipad/id532566885?mt = 8
Sherbrooke Postal Questionnaire (SPQ): http://www.biomedcentral.com/1471–2458/12/69/additional PRISMA-7: http://www.cfp.ca/content/49/8/992.full.pdf
Identification of Seniors At Risk (ISAR) tool: http://www.health.qld.gov.au/hssb/hou/continuityofcare/appendix%20b.pdf

References

1 Lloyd-Sherlock P, McKee M, Ebrahim S, Gorman M, Greengross S, Prince M, Pruchno R, Gutman G, Kirkwood T, O'Neill D, Ferrucci L, Kritchevsky SB, Vellas B: Population ageing and health. Lancet 2012;379:1295–1296.

2 Ward K, Reuben D: Comprehensive geriatric assessment; in UpToDate. 2013. http://www.uptodate.com/contents/comprehensive-geriatric-assessment (accessed May 12, 2014).

3 Rubenstein LZ, Rhee L, Kane RL: The role of geriatric assessment units in caring for the elderly: an analytic review. J Gerontol 1982;37:513–521.

4 Mooney G: What does equity in health mean? World Health Stat Q 1987;40:296–303.

5 Clegg A, Young J, Iliffe S, Rikkert MO, Rockwood K: Frailty in elderly people. Lancet 2013;381:752–762.

6 De Lepeleire J, Iliffe S, Mann E, Degryse JM: Frailty: an emerging concept for general practice. Br J Gen Pract 2009;59:e177–e182.

7 Lacas A, Rockwood K: Frailty in primary care: a review of its conceptualization and implications for practice. BMC Med 2012;10:4.

8 Searle SD, Mitnitski A, Gahbauer EA, Gill TM, Rockwood K: A standard procedure for creating a frailty index. BMC Geriatr 2008;8:24.
9 Theou O, Brothers TD, Mitnitski A, Rockwood K: Operationalization of frailty using eight commonly used scales and comparison of their ability to predict all-cause mortality. J Am Geriatr Soc 2013;61:1537–1551.
10 Romero-Ortuno R: Frailty index in Europeans: association with determinants of health. Geriatr Gerontol Int 2014;14:420–429.
11 Song X, Mitnitski A, Rockwood K: Prevalence and 10-year outcomes of frailty in older adults in relation to deficit accumulation. J Am Geriatr Soc 2010;58: 681–687.
12 Rockwood K, Song X, Mitnitski A: Changes in relative fitness and frailty across the adult lifespan: evidence from the Canadian National Population Health Survey. CMAJ 2011;183:E487–E494.
13 Drubbel I, de Wit NJ, Bleijenberg N, Eijkemans RJ, Schuurmans MJ, Numans ME: Prediction of adverse health outcomes in older people using a frailty index based on routine primary care data. J Gerontol A Biol Sci Med Sci 2013;68:301–308.
14 Fried LP, Tangen CM, Walston J, Newman AB, Hirsch C, Gottdiener J, Seeman T, Tracy R, Kop WJ, Burke G, McBurnie MA: Frailty in older adults: evidence for a phenotype. J Gerontol A Biol Sci Med Sci 2001;56:M146–M156.
15 Eckel SP, Bandeen-Roche K, Chaves PH, Fried LP, Louis TA: Surrogate screening models for the low physical activity criterion of frailty. Aging Clin Exp Res 2011;23:209–216.
16 Romero-Ortuno R, Walsh CD, Lawlor BA, Kenny RA: A frailty instrument for primary care: findings from the Survey of Health, Ageing and Retirement in Europe (SHARE). BMC Geriatr 2010;10:57.
17 Romero-Ortuno R, O'Shea D, Kenny RA: The SHARE frailty instrument for primary care predicts incident disability in a European population-based sample. Qual Prim Care 2011;19:301–309.
18 Romero-Ortuno R: The Frailty Instrument for primary care of the Survey of Health, Ageing and Retirement in Europe predicts mortality similarly to a frailty index based on comprehensive geriatric assessment. Geriatr Gerontol Int 2013;13:497–504.
19 Ntlholang O, Kelly RE, Romero-Ortuno R, Cosgrave S, Kelly D, Crowe M, Collins O, Barry JJ, Cogan L, Hughes G, O'Shea D: The role the frailty syndrome can play in advocacy and resource allocation for our ageing population – findings in a Dublin day hospital. J Frailty Aging 2014;3:21–24.
20 Pialoux T, Goyard J, Lesourd B: Screening tools for frailty in primary health care: a systematic review. Geriatr Gerontol Int 2012;12:189–197.
21 Morley JE, Vellas B, van Kan GA, Anker SD, Bauer JM, Bernabei R, Cesari M, Chumlea WC, Doehner W, Evans J, Fried LP, Guralnik JM, Katz PR, Malmstrom TK, McCarter RJ, Gutierrez Robledo LM, Rockwood K, von Haehling S, Vandewoude MF, Walston J: Frailty consensus: a call to action. J Am Med Dir Assoc 2013;14:392–397.
22 Bandinelli S, Lauretani F, Boscherini V, Gandi F, Pozzi M, Corsi AM, Bartali B, Lova RM, Guralnik JM, Ferrucci L: A randomized, controlled trial of disability prevention in frail older patients screened in primary care: the FRASI study. Design and baseline evaluation. Aging Clin Exp Res 2006;18:359–366.
23 Metzelthin SF, van Rossum E, de Witte LP, Ambergen AW, Hobma SO, Sipers W, Kempen GI: Effectiveness of interdisciplinary primary care approach to reduce disability in community dwelling frail older people: cluster randomised controlled trial. BMJ 2013;347:f5264.
24 Li CM, Chen CY, Li CY, Wang WD, Wu SC: The effectiveness of a comprehensive geriatric assessment intervention program for frailty in community-dwelling older people: a randomized, controlled trial. Arch Gerontol Geriatr 2010;50(suppl 1):S39–S42.
25 Bleijenberg N, Drubbel I, Ten Dam VH, Numans ME, Schuurmans MJ, de Wit NJ: Proactive and integrated primary care for frail older people: design and methodological challenges of the Utrecht primary care PROactive frailty intervention trial (U-PROFIT). BMC Geriatr 2012;12:16.
26 De Lepeleire J, Degryse J, Illiffe S, Mann E, Buntinx F: Family physicians need easy instruments for frailty. Age Ageing 2008;37:484.

Dr. Roman Romero-Ortuno, Lic Med, MSc, MRCP(UK), PhD
Consultant in Care of the Elderly, Department of Medicine for the Elderly, Box 135
Addenbrooke's Hospital, Cambridge University Hospitals NHS Foundation Trust
Hills Road, Cambridge, CB2 0QQ (UK)
E-Mail roman.romero-ortuno@nhs.net

Theou O, Rockwood K (eds): Frailty in Aging. Biological, Clinical and Social Implications.
Interdiscipl Top Gerontol Geriatr. Basel, Karger, 2015, vol 41, pp 95–106 (DOI: 10.1159/000381171)

Hospital Care for Frail Elderly Adults: From Specialized Geriatric Units to Hospital-Wide Interventions

Franka C. Bakker • Marcel G.M. Olde Rikkert

Department of Geriatric Medicine, Radboud University Medical Center, Nijmegen, The Netherlands

Abstract

Much of the acute care provided in hospitals is for elderly people. Frailty is a common clinical condition among these patients. Frail patients are vulnerable to undergoing adverse events, to developing geriatric syndromes and to experiencing functional decline during or due to hospitalization. The strategy for providing specialized geriatric care to these hospitalized frail elderly patients currently consists of care provision either by specialized departments or by specialized teams who adopt comprehensive geriatric assessment. Even so, financial and human resources are insufficient to meet the needs of all hospitalized frail elderly patients who require comprehensive geriatric assessment. New innovative and more efficient geriatric interventions, in which the priorities of the patients themselves should be the main focus, should be developed and implemented, and professionals in all specialties should be educated in applying the fundamentals of geriatric medicine to their frail elderly patients. In the evaluation of such interventions, patient-reported outcomes should play a major role, in addition to the more traditional outcome measures of effectiveness, quality of care and cost-effectiveness.

Never before have so many people lived to grow as old, and with such good prospects in daily functioning, as we do currently [1]. However, with increasing age, the challenges of coping with losses in physical, physiological, cognitive and social functioning accumulate. This so-called *frailty trajectory* becomes particularly visible when elderly people are hospitalized.

Hospital Care for Elders

Much of the acute care provided in hospitals concerns care for elderly people. Patients aged 65 years and older are responsible for more than 40% of all nursing days [2]. An important and very common clinical condition in this patient group is *frailty*. As

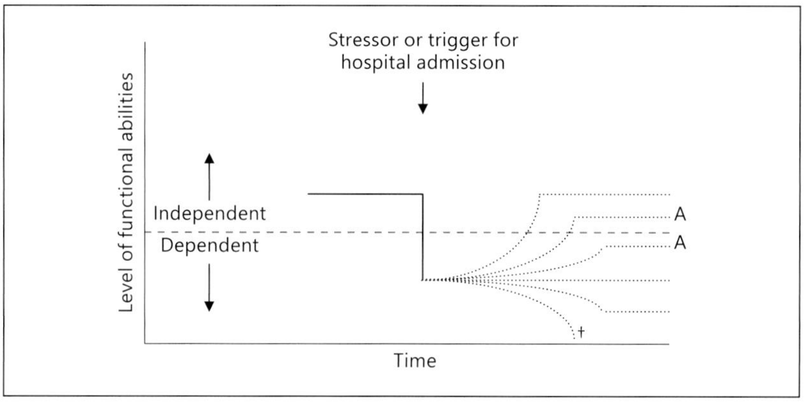

Fig. 1. Frail elderly patients' vulnerability to critical changes in functioning. The dotted lines represent possible trajectories for elderly patients who return or do not return to homeostasis and baseline functioning after a hospital admission. Frail elderly patients may recover their level of independence, either fully or partially, following hospital admission, and this process may be either fast or slow. However, patients may also show no recovery, and even greater decline or death. Slowing down in recovery and an end stage with incomplete recovery are the classical frailty trajectory (A) (Adapted from Clegg et al. [3]).

concisely defined by Clegg et al., frailty develops as a consequence of age-related decline in many physiological systems, which collectively results in vulnerability to sudden health status changes triggered by minor stressor events [3]. Frailty can be seen as a reduced ability to maintain functional equilibrium; certain events or stressors – physical, psychological, social or environmental – may cause disruption of the equilibrium, causing passage below the threshold of independent functioning [4, 5]. Frailty may thus lead to disability under the influence of a stressor [6]. However, great heterogeneity can be distinguished among individual trajectories (see fig. 1).

Prevalence of Frailty

Statistics on the prevalence of frailty among hospitalized patients are scarce, and they are highly dependent on the population included, the definition of frailty used and the assessment methods [7, 8]. For example, among 594 patients aged 65 years and older in an American hospital, the prevalence of both frailty and intermediately frailty was 42% among patients admitted for elective surgery [9]. The researchers used the Fried frailty criteria, which include five physical measures (gait speed, muscle strength, fatigue, weight and exercise). Among 276 patients aged 75 years and older in two Dutch hospitals, the prevalence of frailty varied from 50% of patients in the surgical department to 80% in the internal medicine department to almost 100% in the geriatrics department [10]. The researchers used the Groningen Frailty Indicator and found that most frailty indicators represented the psychosocial scale in addition to the mobility and health scale of the indicator. The large heterogeneity in frailty measures hinders further use and impact on hospital practice, although research on finding common and informative characteristics between frailty measures is increasingly being performed.

Adverse Events

As a consequence of reduced physiological reserves (such as a decline in maximal energy use per unit of time) and failing homeostatic mechanisms (e.g. due to less accurate physiological feedback loops) among frail elderly persons, they are vulnerable to adverse events such as delirium, falls, functional decline, disability, independency, hospitalization, increased care needs, institutionalization and death [3, 7, 11, 12]. However, not only their functional reserves and the acute illness or chronic disease for which they were admitted to the hospital makes them vulnerable for adverse events; a hospital stay in itself is also a risk factor for adverse events [4, 13, 14]. General hospital care processes are often insufficiently adapted to the needs and characteristics of frail elderly patients and therefore may cause unintended injury, resulting in a prolonged hospital stay, disability, or death. These processes include poor management of surgical, medical nondrug and medication procedures as well as inadequate knowledge and education among nurses and physicians regarding care complexities, co-morbidity and frailty [15].

A substantial fraction of adverse events among frail elderly patients is thought to be preventable [14, 15], and especially the development of (new) geriatric syndromes [14], such as mobility impairments, falls, incontinence, polypharmacy, malnutrition, delirium, depression and (other) psychological impairments. A low incidence of hospital-acquired delirium is even said to be an indicator of the quality of hospital care for elderly patients [16]. However, as is the case with monitoring frailty, investigating the incidence and multifaceted causal pathways of adverse events in elderly patients is complex, and statistics are therefore highly dependent on the definition of (preventable) adverse events used and on assessment methods, e.g. incidence rates range from 5.3% up to 60% [14].

Hospital-Associated Disability

Nevertheless, disability is often described as one of the most important (consequences of) adverse events of hospital admission among frail elderly inpatients, as it results in a poor prognosis for independent functioning, increased use of healthcare services and mortality. The quality of hospital care probably plays an important role both in the success rate of recovery of the functional loss that occurred (shortly) before admission due to the illness, leading to hospital admission, and in prevention of additional functional decline during hospitalization [4]. These negative effects of hospitalization on functional performance were already described decades ago as the 'hazards of hospitalization of the elderly' [17].

By definition, hospital-associated disability is the development of a new disability in activities of daily living (ADL) at hospital discharge that was not present before the onset of the acute illness. These include disabilities regarding the six most basic ADL: bathing, dressing, rising from bed or a chair, using the toilet, eating, and walking across a room. It is estimated that at least 30% of hospitalized patients aged 70 years and older develop hospital-associated disability [4, 13]. Among frail elderly patients this is even worse as – due to the multifactorial nature of frailty – a change in health status often leads to a cascade of negative events toward functional decline [3]. This is based on the fact that elderly persons face age- or disease-related changes in many (interrelated) organ systems, which precede frailty or vulnerability to stressors [3, 6, 17].

For example, changes in the musculoskeletal system may cause reduced muscle strength, leading to immobility. Restricted mobility during a hospital stay due to bed rest or all kinds of barriers to improving physical activity may further reduce muscle strength, bone density and mobility, possibly leading to deconditioning, falls and fractures, and/or (increased) dependency. Changes in the integumentary system and digestive system may cause altered thirst and nutrition, leading to a risk of dehydration and malnutrition. A restricted hospital diet and physical and social barriers to eating/drinking in bed, possibly in addition to disease-associated dehydration, may increase this risk further. Fragile skin in combination with bed rest increases the risk of pressure sores and infections. Changes in the nervous system and brain may increase the risk of cognitive impairments, and in addition, changes in the sensory system may cause people to be confused when in a strange and isolated environment. As such, numerous pathways related to inadequate hospital care for frail elderly are observed in clinical practice [17]. These pathways are dependent on many different physiological mechanisms as well as a lack of support within the hospital to administer timely preventive activities.

Organization of Care

Therefore, a very important question for judging the quality of hospital care may be whether frail elderly patients develop new or more severe psychological or functional impairment, leading to (further) loss of independent functioning. Figure 2 shows that overall, a few categories of hospital processes may be the main indicators of whether adequate care for hospitalized frail elderly patients is being provided. These indicators include the engaging or restricting characteristics of the physical hospital environment, (a lack of) knowledge of and attention to frailty among nurses and physicians, tailored patient-centered care, prolonged bed rest and the use of physical constraints. This is in contrast to encouragement of mobilization and independent performance

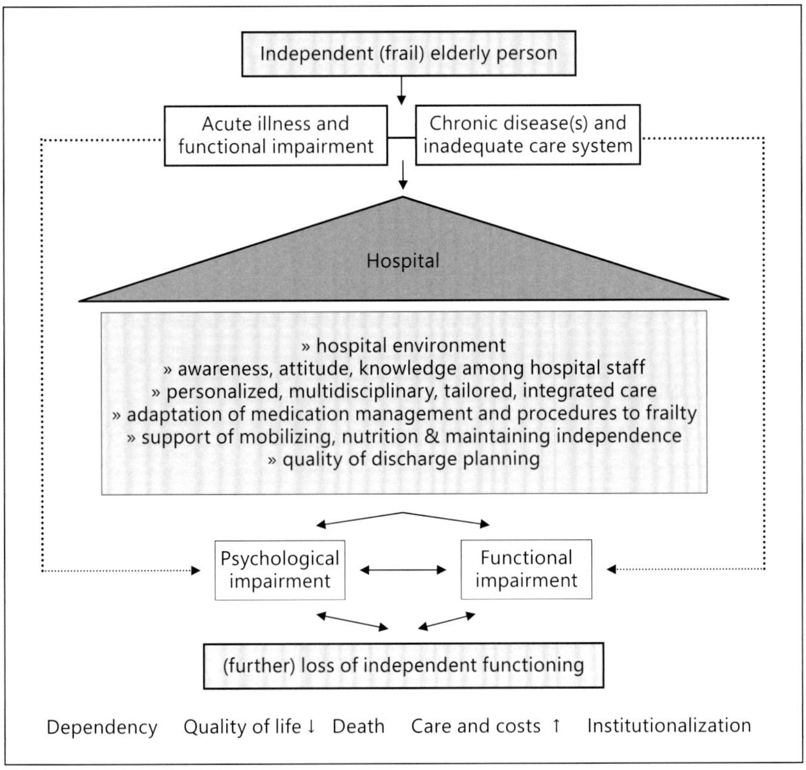

Fig. 2. Interaction of patient- and hospital-related factors, causing (increased) functional impairment in frail elderly inpatients. In addition to the frailty status of a patient and the severity of his or her illnesses, hospital care processes that are not adapted to individual needs and common changes in organ systems in frail elderly patients may cause adverse events and hospital-associated disability (Adapted from Lafont et al. [13]).

of ADL, frailty-adapted medication management and care procedures, and high-quality discharge planning [4, 13]. It is assumed that hospital-acquired delirium, functional decline and frailty can be prevented, delayed or treated if appropriate interventions and care are provided adequately [6, 18].

Specialized Geriatric Interventions

The geriatric medicine specialty provides tailored care, with performance of a comprehensive geriatric assessment (CGA) as a basic principle. CGA is defined as a 'multidimensional interdisciplinary diagnostic process focused on determining a frail elderly person's medical, psychological and functional capability in order to develop a coordinated and integrated plan for treatment and long-term follow-up' [19, 20]. It can be delivered either by geriatric hospital departments with specialized staff or by specialized geriatrics teams across various hospital departments. For the first model,

CGA has been proven to benefit frail older patients, who are alive and living in their home after a certain period of follow-up, and results in a shorter length of stay, fewer readmissions, less functional decline, fewer iatrogenic complications, and possibly more cost-effectiveness, but the benefit is less clear and more controversial for geriatrics teams [20–26]. For both models, a precondition for effectiveness is that CGA should be combined with management and intervention strategies, also referred to as geriatric evaluation and management. The basic principles of CGA and the two general models of providing it (via departments and teams) are also represented in several other hospital-wide interventions to improve care for hospitalized frail elderly inpatients, e.g. the Hospital Elder Life Program and the Nurses Improving Care for Health System Elders program [26].

The success and effectiveness of CGA and subsequent interventions are thought to be dependent on numerous factors [19–22, 24, 26]:

- healthcare and financing systems, e.g. no fragmentation, with collaborative provision of follow-up services;
- high quality of coordination and continuity of care among healthcare professionals and institutions, e.g. follow-up and provision of rehabilitative services;
- availability of sufficient trained professionals, i.e. a well-functioning assessment team intensively involved in care processes;
- success of geriatrics projects in the past and the support of important actors (e.g. managers, board of directors, medical specialists);
- perceived sense of urgency and priority for geriatric medicine among hospital staff and adoption of geriatric care principles, e.g. modifying behaviors and adhering to interventions;
- quality of evidence gathered from original proof-of-concept studies, e.g. sample size and study design;
- heterogeneity among patient populations, patient targeting, complexity of interventions, study settings and evaluation methods.

With regard to these factors, there is an extreme amount of heterogeneity among the hospital interventions targeting the frail elderly population, and there still is no clear evidence-based practice, though these services 'form the very heart and soul of geriatrics' (Cohen [27]). This causes problems in answering the who, what, where, when, why and how questions in geriatrics management within daily practice and scientific evaluation. The key for successful interventions probably lies in the answers to primary questions like the following: Which patients need CGA? Which professionals should be carrying out the intervention? What should CGA consist of exactly? Where and at what moment should it be performed? What are the goals? How and with what intensity should it be done to ensure effectiveness?

Remarkably, the importance of these factors and questions has not changed much during the past decades. The search for how to improve hospital care for frail elderly patients across all departments in the continuously changing and modernizing hospital environment is continuing.

Geriatric and Frailty Evaluation

CGA improves diagnostic accuracy due to the comprehensive and multidisciplinary perspective of the evaluation, and thus, its value is not particularly questioned by healthcare professionals, management staff or healthcare insurers. However, it is considered time consuming and costly, with the consequence that hospitals are forced to ensure that only those patients who will really benefit from the investment and show the added value both quantitatively and qualitatively receive CGA and indicated interventions.

Patient Targeting, Screening, Risk Assessment, Case Finding, Triage, and Referral

Therefore, instruments have been developed to figure out which elderly patients should receive additional attention and interventions to prevent hospital-acquired complications and (further) functional deterioration [28, 29]. These include, for example, the following:

- Identification of Seniors at Risk;
- Hospital Admission Risk Profile;
- Triage Risk Screening Tool;
- Score Hospitalier d'Evaluation du Risque de Perte d'Autonomie;
- Brief Risk Identification for Geriatric Health Tool;
- Hospital Elder Life Program screening criteria.

Screening items may include, for instance, age, physical parameters, laboratory markers, hospitalization history, polypharmacy, geriatric conditions or co-morbidities, functional impairments and social problems. However, as for the definition for frailty, no uniform screening instrument appropriately identifies all patients at risk for functional decline [28]. Therefore, although screening may help to identify those patients who need additional interventions the most, the pros and cons of instruments should be considered when choosing an instrument.

The instruments mentioned above assess the risk of adverse events or triage for targeting an intervention and are not explicitly used for frailty screening (e.g. Fried phenotype [30]) or frailty assessment (e.g. Rockwood frailty index [30]). Nonetheless, interest in targeting based on frailty is increasing among medical disciplines. Links between frailty and other diseases are being made, and studies determining the predictive value of frailty (indices/scales) for patient outcomes are being performed more often. It is a challenge for all medical specialties to deliver the proper multifactorial interventions based on screening or assessments in order to meet the needs of the changing and aging hospital patient population, in addition to geriatrics departments and specialized geriatrics teams, which have already existed for years. The needs and expectations of frail elderly inpatients are different from those of the general hospital population and therefore require a different approach in hospital management and processes. As there are no clear frailty screening instruments, creating prospective (Rockwood) frailty indices from patient files should be easily accomplishable, as many important and informative data are already being gathered from patients. A medical history can, for example, be based on the EASY-Care instrument. This is an instrument that structures the first broad assessment in an easy way for a nonspecialist in geriatrics and that is now widely used in primary and community care as a standardized CGA instrument for holistic and preventive care [31].

Geriatric and Frailty Management

Although demographic, economic and epidemiological changes have been foreseen for years and although medical innovations have strongly improved treatment possibilities, particularly for the elderly population, many developments in the healthcare delivery system that do not fit the needs of the growing group of frail elderly patients with multiple chronic diseases, who are coming from complex care environments, have occurred. These developments include, for example, a reduction in length of stay; decentralization and concentration of care, including increased specialization and high-tech hospital care; and application of quality measures and benchmarks developed for disease-specific purposes. Hospital services not only need to innovate but also need to take into account evidence regarding frailty and frailty-related interventions while doing so.

For example, shortening of hospital length of stay increases the importance of continuation of geriatric care after hospital discharge in order to ensure optimal rehabilitation to the desired functional level (fig. 1). However, it is often extremely complex to design efficient and effective cooperation and follow-up models for primary care or other healthcare facilities/providers. Therefore, improving transfers from hospital to home or other care facilities/providers, as already repeatedly pointed out by researchers in geriatric interventions, remains an important recommendation for the future. Currently, important and promising initiatives for creating care networks arise, e.g. in the Dutch National Care for the Elderly Program, in which the value of telemedicine and e-health for the frail elderly population with complex care needs is also being further explored.

In addition, the current models of geriatric care supplement other medical specialties in the process of providing integrated care for frail elderly patients with complex needs. In these models – which, for example, are used in oncology, trauma surgery, emergency wards, orthopedics, and cardiology – medical skills in geriatrics and individual training are offered to residents, but actual care provision remains dependent on nonspecialists in geriatrics. In rapidly changing and complex hospital environments, priority setting may be different between medical specialists. Therefore, the skills and competencies needed in geriatrics teams for collaboration and for establishment of a sense of urgency about changing hospital care for the general frail elderly population among medical specialists are becoming increasingly important now. Besides the changing competences among geriatrics specialists in advocating policies for geriatric, preferably everybody should fundamentally rethink hospital service provision for frail elderly patients, as elderly patients account for 40–50% of all bed days, so their care concerns almost all medical specialties. In this transition toward hospital-wide safe and efficient care, efforts such as senior- or elder-friendly hospitals are encouraging systems, processes and a physical environment that are supported by elder-friendly hospital policies, procedures and social climates [32, 33]. Another example is the development of hospital care pathways for elderly patients, in which geriatric medicine is more often incorporated with other medical specialties on their request, such as in co-management models in orthopedics (hip fractures), cardiology, oncology and emergency medicine. Educating professionals in the physiology, recognition and adaptation of care in the domain of frailty is a first priority to improve hospital care for elderly patients, before one can successfully implement other models of care. An interesting example going in the direction of education is the Nurses Improving Care for Health System Elders model.

Another trend in healthcare is continuous quality improvement; benchmarking; and the use of quality indicators as part of hospital performance, such as the Assessing Care of Vulnerable Elders quality indicators [34]. However, again, the outcomes of such process measures are dependent on the quality indicator sets used, the setting and the population (case mix). In addition, monitoring such routine administrative data is valuable and can direct hospital management in the development of quality improvement efforts, but for individual nurses and physicians, insight into the actual effect on patients' outcomes may better stimulate adaption of care to the needs of their patients. A growing field of interest is that of patient-reported outcome measures (PROMs). PROMs may increasingly be gathered from and within electronic patient records and provides valuable information for clinicians, hospital management, patients and researchers [35, 36]. If frailty indices could be prospectively generated from electronic patient records, together with PROMS, it would be possible to provide the ability to properly target interventions and to monitor and compare outcomes for frail elderly patients. The challenge for the future would be to develop an appropriate, standardized, interpretable and workable set of PROMs and objectified effectiveness outcome measures for this patient population, in which the patients' perspectives are truly represented. These patients may be very different from other patient groups due to their frailty status and trajectory of rehabilitation, i.e. not limited to classical outcomes (e.g. mortality, morbidity and functional performance) and healthcare utilization. Satisfaction with care and wellbeing throughout a hospital stay are probably increasingly important as the life expectancy for frail elderly persons decreases. This notion of shifted weight of outcomes is still only preliminarily explored in clinical practice and science. Additionally, shared goal setting may result in new responsive outcome measures, though goal attainment scaling is also difficult to implement in geriatric patients with cognitive decline.

Research Dilemmas

In developing innovative evidence-based frailty-oriented hospital services, researchers face various methodological challenges. Many difficulties exist in finding the proper evaluation methods for this complex subject, which focuses on extremely heterogeneous patient groups, settings, interventions and research possibilities. Therefore, innovative research methods are also needed. The classical (cluster) randomized controlled trial often does not fit the complex nature of changes in our complex hospital healthcare, which can often only be partly completely preplanned or predicted.

Currently, the focus on process and quality-control evaluation increases when trying to deal with the complexity of the evaluation of innovative and multicomponent interventions, such as interventions to improve hospital care for frail elderly patients. Process evaluation may provide more detailed insight into the who, what, where, when, why and how questions. It describes how an intervention and study were conducted for a specific practice and for a specific targeted frail population and thereby may aid the development, evaluation, interpretation and dissemination of practices. However, no standardized formats for how to perform process evaluation exist, causing difficulties in valuing the findings within process evaluations [37], although landmark papers on process evaluations are increasingly being published.

Another trend is the performance of pragmatic studies in order to narrow the gap between research and practice. Pragmatic studies are designed to determine whether a program works under usual conditions, as opposed to ideal conditions in a randomized controlled trial. Pragmatic measures [38], such as electronically monitored PROMs, may be more appropriate for use in innovative intervention studies including frail elderly patients and in complex environments such as the always-changing dynamic hospital environment. Pragmatic measures can be monitored continuously and thereby may facilitate the flexible evaluation of interventions, outcomes and resources in addition to or instead of monitoring the fixed and limited study measures in a static study design. These measures can be of value for researchers, policy makers and practitioners and may eventually guide us to lean, cost-effective hospital-wide practices for frail elderly patients, as their care will always need to be provided from a more or less generalist approach, with a focus on setting priorities for offering healthcare interventions. As long as the hospital-wide answer to the challenge of frailty is lacking, reporting of purely scientific results and studies on process measures is required, in addition to access to the results of quality improvement projects, which may not qualify for scientific publication per se. This will help us to develop evidence-based and practice-based hospital services for frail elderly patients, which are also necessary for the hospital to survive as the most important healthcare provider for all.

Concluding Remarks

The strategy for providing specialized geriatric care to hospitalized frail elderly patients currently consists of care provision either by specialized departments or by specialized teams using CGA. However, these services are insufficient to meet the needs of all hospitalized frail elderly patients, who are increasingly becoming the core business of many medical specialties. New innovative geriatric interventions, in which the priorities of the patients themselves should be the main focus, should be developed and implemented, and professionals should be educated in applying the fundamentals of geriatric medicine to their frail elderly patients. In the evaluation of such interventions, patient-reported outcomes can play a major role, in addition to the more traditional outcome measures of effectiveness, quality of care and cost-effectiveness, which probably should be fewer and should be selected more carefully. Current developments force hospital staff to offer frailty-based practices to all frail elderly patients, for whom the hospital stay is a short but highly intensive and crucial phase in their frailty trajectories.

References

1 Christensen K, Thinggaard M, Oksuzyan A, et al: Physical and cognitive functioning of people older than 90 years: a comparison of two Danish cohorts born 10 years apart. Lancet 2013;382:1507–1513.
2 Buie VC, Owings MF, DeFrances CJ, et al: National Hospital Discharge Survey: 2006 Annual Summary. Hyattsville, MD, National Center for Health Statistics, 2010.
3 Clegg A, Young J, Iliffe S, et al: Frailty in elderly people. Lancet 2013;381:752–762.
4 Covinsky KE, Pierluissi E, Johnston CB: Hospitalization-associated disability: 'She was probably able to ambulate, but I'm not sure'. JAMA 2011;306:1782–1793.
5 McMillan GJ, Hubbard RE: Frailty in older inpatients: what physicians need to know. QJM 2012;105:1059–1065.
6 Heuberger RA: The frailty syndrome: a comprehensive review. J Nutr Gerontol Geriatr 2011;30:315–368.
7 Sternberg SA, Wershof Schwartz A, Karunananthan S, et al: The identification of frailty: a systematic literature review. J Am Geriatr Soc 2011;59:2129–2138.
8 Partridge JS, Harari D, Dhesi JK: Frailty in the older surgical patient: a review. Age Ageing 2012;41:142–147.
9 Makary MA, Segev DL, Pronovost PJ, et al: Frailty as a predictor of surgical outcomes in older patients. J Am Coll Surg 2010;210:901–908.
10 Andela RM, Dijkstra A, Slaets JP, et al: Prevalence of frailty on clinical wards: description and implications. Int J Nurs Pract 2010;16:14–19.
11 Ruiz M, Cefalu C, Reske T: Frailty syndrome in geriatric medicine. Am J Med Sci 2012;344:395–398.
12 Quinlan N, Marcantonio ER, Inouye SK, et al: Vulnerability: the crossroads of frailty and delirium. J Am Geriatr Soc 2011;59(suppl 2):S262–S268.
13 Lafont C, Gérard S, Voisin T, et al: Reducing 'iatrogenic disability' in the hospitalized frail elderly. J Nutr Health Aging 2011;15:645–660.
14 Long SJ, Brown KF, Ames D, et al: What is known about adverse events in older medical hospital inpatients? A systematic review of the literature. Int J Qual Health Care 2013;25:542–554.
15 Merten H, Zegers M, de Bruijne MC, et al: Scale, nature, preventability and causes of adverse events in hospitalised older patients. Age Ageing 2013;42:87–93.
16 Inouye SK: Delirium: a barometer for quality of hospital care. Hosp Pract (1995) 2001;36:15–16.
17 Creditor MC: Hazards of hospitalization of the elderly. Ann Intern Med 1993;118:219–223.
18 Siddiqi N, House AO, Holmes JD: Occurrence and outcome of delirium in medical in-patients: a systematic literature review. Age Ageing 2006;35:350–364.

19 Rubenstein LZ, Stuck AE, Siu AL, et al: Impacts of geriatric evaluation and management programs on defined outcomes: overview of the evidence. J Am Geriatr Soc 1991;39(9 Pt 2):8S-18S.
20 Ellis G, Whitehead MA, Robinson D, et al: Comprehensive geriatric assessment for older adults admitted to hospital: meta-analysis of randomised controlled trials. BMJ 2011;343:d6553.
21 Baztan JJ, Suárez-García FM, López-Arrieta J, et al: Effectiveness of acute geriatric units on functional decline, living at home, and case fatality among older patients admitted to hospital for acute medical disorders: meta-analysis. BMJ 2009;338:b50.
22 Van Craen K, Braes T, Wellens N, et al: The effectiveness of inpatient geriatric evaluation and management units: a systematic review and meta-analysis. J Am Geriatr Soc 2010;58:83–92.
23 Fox MT, Persaud M, Maimets I, et al: Effectiveness of acute geriatric unit care using acute care for elders components: a systematic review and meta-analysis. J Am Geriatr Soc 2012;60:2237–2245.
24 Deschodt M, Flamaing J, Haentjens P, et al: Impact of geriatric consultation teams on clinical outcome in acute hospitals: a systematic review and meta-analysis. BMC Med 2013;11:48.
25 Fox MT, Sidani S, Persaud M, et al: Acute care for elders components of acute geriatric unit care: systematic descriptive review. J Am Geriatr Soc 2013; 61:939–946.
26 Bakker FC, Robben SH, Olde Rikkert MG: Effects of hospital-wide interventions to improve care for frail older inpatients: a systematic review. BMJ Qual Saf 2011;20:680–691.
27 Cohen HJ: Commentary on: Impacts of geriatric evaluation and management programs on defined outcomes; overview of the evidence. J Am Geriatr Soc 1991;39:8S–16S.
28 De Saint-Hubert M, Schoevaerdts D, Cornette P, et al: Predicting functional adverse outcomes in hospitalized older patients: a systematic review of screening tools. J Nutr Health Aging 2010;14:394–399.
29 Beaton K, Grimmer K: Tools that assess functional decline: systematic literature review update. Clin Interv Aging 2013;8:485–494.
30 Cesari M, Gambassi G, van Kan GA, et al: The frailty phenotype and the frailty index: different instruments for different purposes. Age Ageing 2014;43: 10–12.
31 Olde-Rikkert MG, Long JF, Philp I: Development and evidence base of a new efficient assessment instrument for international use by nurses in community settings with older people. Int J Nurs Stud 2013; 50:1180–1183.
32 Parke B, Stevenson L: Creating an elder-friendly hospital. Healthc Manage Forum 1999;12:45–48.
33 Parke B, Hunter KF, Bostrom AM, et al: Identifying modifiable factors to improve quality for older adults in hospital: a scoping review. Int J Older People Nurs 2014;9:8–24.
34 Askari M, Wierenga PC, Eslami S, et al: Assessing quality of care of elderly patients using the ACOVE quality indicator set: a systematic review. PLoS One 2011;6:e28631.
35 Wu AW, Kharrazi H, Boulware LE, et al: Measure once, cut twice – adding patient-reported outcome measures to the electronic health record for comparative effectiveness research. J Clin Epidemiol 2013; 66(8 suppl):S12–S20.
36 Snyder CF, Jensen RE, Segal JB, et al: Patient-reported outcomes (PROs): putting the patient perspective in patient-centered outcomes research. Med Care 2013;51(8 suppl 3):S73–S79.
37 Bakker FC, Persoon A, Reelick MF, et al: Evidence from multicomponent interventions: value of process evaluations. J Am Geriatr Soc 2013;61:844–845.
38 Glasgow RE, Riley WT: Pragmatic measures: what they are and why we need them. Am J Prev Med 2013;45:237–243.

Prof. Dr. Marcel G.M. Olde Rikkert
Department of Geriatric Medicine 925
Radboud University Medical Center
PO Box 9101, 6500 HB Nijmegen (The Netherlands)
E-Mail Marcel.OldeRikkert@radboudumc.nl

Theou O, Rockwood K (eds): Frailty in Aging. Biological, Clinical and Social Implications.
Interdiscipl Top Gerontol Geriatr. Basel, Karger, 2015, vol 41, pp 107–120 (DOI: 10.1159/000381200)

Frailty and Mobility

Eamonn Eeles[a, b] · Nancy Low Choy[b, c]

[a]Internal Medicine Services, The Prince Charles Hospital and [b]The Prince Charles Hospital, The University of Queensland, Chermside, and [c]School of Physiotherapy, Faculty of Health Sciences, Australian Catholic University, Banyo, Qld., Australia

Abstract

Frailty represents a state of heightened vulnerability. Mobility impairment contributes to the construct of frailty and channels adverse events. While mobility disorder is universal at a high burden of frailty, neither mobility nor balance dysfunction is sufficient to fully define frailty. Frailty represents proximity to complex system failure, with higher-order disturbance, such as mobility and balance disturbance, as a consequence. Impairment of mobility and balance is a common manifestation of illness in the frail individual and is therefore a sensitive marker of acute disease, putatively also in delirium. Clinical measurement of mobility and balance should be prioritized. Consequently, assessment tools, such as the de Morton Mobility Index and the Hierarchical Assessment of Balance and Mobility, are being explored, with the sensitivity of the latter illustrated in the acute hospital setting. Walking with speed and under dual/multi-task conditions better differentiates healthier and frail ambulant adults, providing a basis for screening older adults for pre-emptive interventions. Specific mobility and balance interventions reduce falls risk. However, patients with dementia walk too fast for their level of frailty, creating an ethical dimension to rehabilitation and risk. Overall, there is no need for reduced mobility to reinforce the frailty stereotype; both are potentially modifiable and amenable to intervention strategies.

'The length of his walk uniformly made the length of his writing. If shut up in the house, he did not write at all.' – Ralph Waldo Emerson

Frailty is a syndrome that confers vulnerability on older adults. Mobility disturbance contributes to the burden of frailty and influences the level of independence and adverse events. Upright bipedalism is a uniquely human endeavor achieved only through impressive central nervous system (CNS) integration that is commensurate with higher-order function. The dividend of independent mobility is offset by intrinsic threats to mobility in low-threshold frailty states in which the hazards of falls and dependency are imminent. Specific transition states in mobility are most prevalent in frail older adults, involving peripheral and central changes, with notable impacts when cognitive deficits and/or dementia present. Dual tasks pose specific challenges as reduced attention control emerges, and careless gait in dementia confers specific challenges to mobility, with falls as a frequent consequence.

On the simplest level, impairment in mobility may appear to equate to the mental construct of frailty. At the population level, immobility may indeed be associated with submaximal levels of frailty and the implication of functional and cognitive decline. With greater physical robustness, the interrelationship between frailty and mobility is less clear. It is not hard to posit that at the individual level, a person who is frail but independent may be rendered entirely dependent on the whim of decreases in mobility. The two entities therefore have huge clinical significance in the field of elder care. Acute geriatrics, orthogeriatrics, rehabilitation and falls clinics often represent the clash of reduced mobility and frailty with social, economic and personal ramifications.

This chapter explores multiple themes related to balance and mobility. The levels of frailty at which mobility is affected, the mechanistic relationship between frailty and mobility and the syndromes and conditions that modulate this relationship are first considered. These principles are followed by considerations of frailty and mobility within acute care of older adults, measurement of frailty and mobility and the implications for rehabilitation. Some of the ethical dilemmas that arise and the attitudes influenced by the interaction of frailty with mobility are discussed. These insights offer a conceptual basis for screening, prevention and intervention strategies that lead into chapter 12, on 'Frailty and Rehabilitation'.

How Frailty and Mobility Relate

Falls can be understood as a black swan event in a frail adult. Difficult to predict, falls are often subject to flawed rationalization. Adverse consequences of significant magnitude follow: loss of confidence, decreased mobility, deconditioning, social withdrawal and fear of falling can be overwhelming, even before the traumatic sequelae are calculated. For a frail individual, a co-existent gait or balance disorder precedes such a fall. The mechanism by which this occurs is partially inevitable, due to impaired locomotion and the reduced adaptability of the person to falling, which is akin to walking a tightrope without a stabilizer. It is also believed that manifestation of failure in a complex system is represented by disturbance in higher-order function. Consciousness, divided attention, and mobility are the higher-order attributes whose dysfunction is expressed as geriatric syndromes. Mobility, if serving as a marker of complex system integrity, should also carry prognostic significance, such as the ability to predict falls or mortality. Certainly, in-hospital immobility has been shown to be associated with an in-hospital mortality rate of nearly 50% compared with universal survival and discharge for patients achieving full mobility and balance [1]. The improvement of mobility becomes a reasonable goal and an indicator of wider system resumption of complex system order.

Mobility also qualifies as a higher-order function through the multi-modal and polysensory neuronal integration of what is a definitively specialized, kinematically exacting yet almost infinitely variable, and evolutionarily distinct function. Clearly, disturbed mobility in a frail individual, particularly if an acute episode presents that is not accounted for by a middle- or lower-order gait disorder, denotes complex system failure. Thus, the approach to understanding the problem should be less through the prism of Newton's third law (a reduction in mobility must be due to a problem with the apparatus of mobility, or the legs) and more through the paradigm of system entropy, with disorder across the macrostate and notable dysfunction at the apex (the CNS). As there is built-in redundancy within complex systems, it takes multiple deficits and erosion of functional mechanisms before disorder and higher-order dysfunction are realized. Hence, increased energy from the system of management, or comprehensive geriatric assessment, must be invested to salvage order from disorder. It is likely that a threshold of resilience must be breached before actualization of higher-order dysfunction occurs in the form of the frail individual. Therefore, diminished mobility in the frail person may be the consequence of locomotor problems or a manifestation of complex system failure, with a fall representing a disruptive consequence.

There is a clear relationship between frailty and mobility: impairment in balance and mobility is universal at high frailty burden (frailty index (FI) >0.45) and leads to functional decline [2]. However, mobility and balance are insufficient to fully define frailty [3], in keeping with the tenet that multiple systems are implicated in frailty. This makes intuitive sense. Despite the limitations brought about by locomotor immobility, there are potential gains made through compensation, specialization, adaptation and relearning that may offset mobility impairment and restore independence. However, when mobility impairment arises in the context of frailty, then activity limitation and participation restriction inevitably follow. Mobility impairment can be seen as a canary in the mine of complex system function, with gait disturbance serving an early warning of failure in a frail individual.

Specific Mobility Disorders and Frailty

Gait disorders are conventionally divided into higher-, middle- and lower-order disturbances [4]. Higher-level gait classification unifies the phenotypic and neuroanatomical bases for an array of gait dyspraxias in which there are abnormalities of the highest sensorimotor circuitry. Middle-order gait disorders represent problems in basic sensorimotor systems from the brain to the spine, whereas lower-order disorders include disturbance from below the level of the spinal cord to the effector organ. Coupled with the hierarchy of gait disorders and their specific etiologies is a presumption of increased disability and, in many instances, frailty. However, there are few data to specifically test this premise. Indeed, the Fried phenotype excluded Parkinson's disease from the original frailty phenotype studies [5]. The deficit accumulation model is inclusive of gait disorders captured as a deficit in order to derive an FI. Nevertheless, frailty has not been specifically described for individual mobility disorders.

The Consequences of Impaired Mobility and Frailty

As we have argued, robustness, the antithesis of frailty, may buffer against the consequences of immobility. By contrast, quality-adjusted health diminishes greatly when frailty and impaired mobility co-exist. The addition of poverty, social exclusion and/or a lack of environmental adaptation often makes independent living untenable when mobility is threatened. Impaired mobility may interact in a nonlinear fashion with other functions, worsening frailty-related attributes when they were not previously apparent, e.g. during dressing or grooming. Even if care is provided within the right setting, the direct consequences of a sessile existence, such as the risk of pressure sores, urinary tract infections and even stigmatization, may continue. However, the adverse consequences of frailty and diminished mobility are not inevitable, and outcomes can be optimized.

Frailty and Mobility within Acute Care

Archetypal symptoms of acute illness are frequently missing in frail older patients. Instead, geriatric syndromes, such as impaired mobility and balance, are the commonest manifestations of acute disease in this population. The etiological factors shared across the syndromes are represented by the problems that older patients present with: iatrogenesis (due to prescribed or over-the-counter medications or medications plus alcohol), cardiac problems, infection, metabolic problems, some other illness, or some combination of these. This is often a trap for the unwary practitioner. Linear causality has assisted modern medicine greatly but may not apply so readily to the outlined scenario of complex system failure. Acute mobility disturbance in a frail patient is therefore insufficiently characterized, as are the causes. Mobility and balance impairment is therefore a sensitive, if nonspecific, indicator of acuity in frail patients. If mobility and balance represent system integrity, then their monitoring also provides a way of tracking physiological progress and response to treatment.

What is needed is an understanding of the importance of and an openness to embracing the conceptual framework for acute mobility decline without neglecting to recognize when traditional evaluation serves us well. There are implications for both processes of care and patient outcomes: the prioritization of mobility assessment and the ability to conduct serial evaluation may also liberate prognostic information. Mobility must be actively nurtured in each patient, elevating the status of functional mobility to a primary goal for the multi-disciplinary team (MDT). Accordingly, measurement of mobility is paramount, with the right choice of tool for the right setting required. We propose such tools in our consideration of clinical measures.

Frailty and Mobility in Dementia

Frailty, cognitive impairment and impaired mobility form an unholy alliance. Frail elderly patients with dementia walk too fast for their level of frailty [6, 7]. Potential factors include frontal lobe disinhibition and a lack of insight into risk. The high risk of falls in dementia may be partially explained by the loss of control of gait velocity, gait variability, slower reaction time, reduced functional mobility and depression. It should also be noted that mobility disturbance may be key to the diagnosis of dementia subtypes, with characteristic features observed in vascular dementia (hemiparetic gait or higher-order gait disturbance), Parkinson's disease with dementia (festinant gait), and Parkinson's plus syndromes (postural instability). Gait variability suggests a higher frailty state, an association that may be mediated by early higher-order gait dysfunction in dementia [7]. Cognitive distraction may increase imbalance in frail individuals [8]. It may not be realistic to promote functional mobility in patients who are in a residential high-care setting with dementia, and indeed, in some instances, the contrary may be required. An inverse relationship between mobility and falls has been documented in these settings, with those requiring supervision most at risk of a fall [9]. However, just because a patient is unable to enjoy full mobility does not preclude the benefits of physical activity. Transfer activities involving sitting and standing may be feasible ways of maintaining functional lower limb strength in high-care facilities, preserving physical fitness and potentially reducing carer burden [10]. At a certain juncture, mobility confers a direct imminent threat to personal safety (through fall and fracture or adverse interaction with fellow man). Therefore, the issue of restraint arises when refractory behavioral and psychiatric symptoms of dementia arise. Leaving the thankfully largely historical matter of physical restraint aside, the option of chemical restraint arises. In our experience, the risk of physical danger needs to be weighed carefully against the imposition on autonomy and dignity. Of course, mobility from a dementia patient's perspective is often taken to mean driving. While not covered in this chapter, driving remains a challenging extended function in frailty, for which the will to continue is often only rivaled by the risks that it may present.

Why Mobility Must Be Disturbed in Delirium

Patients with delirium are also frail [11]. If frail individuals who already have mobility or attentional deficits experience delirium, then it is rational that mobility will suffer. There is more to this relationship than just an exaggeration of a predisposition.

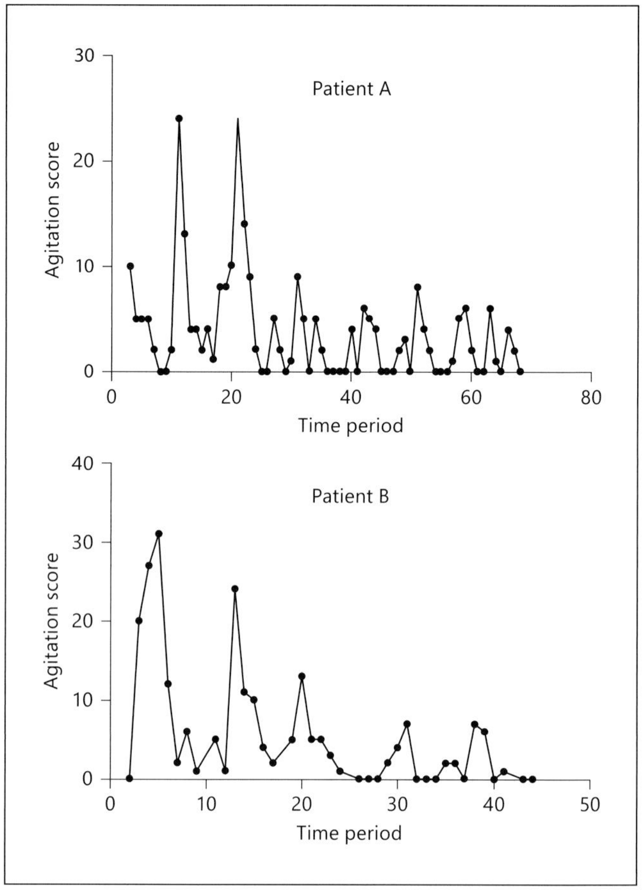

Fig. 1. The patterns of agitation in delirium that improves (patient A) and in pre-terminal delirium (patient B) over time. Each time period refers to an epoch of 6 hours. The agitation profiles are indistinguishable, and the distinction between the two types of delirium is observed in mobility (see fig. 2).

Consciousness embodies all waking thoughts. Disturbance of consciousness is integral to delirium, with every domain of human thought or behavior interrupted in (the totality of descriptions of) delirium. By extension, there can be no expression of self-agency, mobility included, within the sphere of consciousness that is not also impacted by delirium.

Mobility and consciousness also share the pedestal of higher-order function, and integrity is impaired during stress or illness in a frail person. However, delirium remains a persistent problem. Herein, the assessment of mobility and balance offers diagnostic and monitoring insights. It is conceivable that mobility and balance fluctuate in the same way that attention wavers, and tracking both may map disease progress. Unpublished but recently presented data suggest that patients who improve following delirium differ in mobility from those with pre-terminal delirium (see fig. 1, 2).

Future research should focus on this area by investigating the utility of mobility assessment in delirium.

		BL	Example 1 days 1–6						Example 2 days 1–6					
	Recorder's Initials	EE	EE	EE	EE	EE	EE	EE	EE	EE	EE	EE	EE	EE
	Date Assessed (DD)	–14	15	16	17	18	19	20	15	16	17	18	19	20
	(MM)	1	1	1	1	1	1	1	1	1	1	1	1	1
Score	**BALANCE**													
21	Stable ambulation	15												15
14	Stable dynamic standing												14	
10	Stable static standing		10		10				10		10			
7	Stable dynamic sitting			7		7				7		7		
5	Stable static sitting						5							
0	Impaired static sitting							0						
	TRANSFERS													
18	Independent + vigorous													
16	Independent													
14	Independent but slow	14												14
12	1 person standby		12						12		12		12	
11	1 person minimum assistance			11	11					11		11		
7	1 person assist					7								
3	2 person assist						3							
0	Total lift							0						
	MOBILITY													
28	Unlimited, vigorous													
26	Unlimited													
25	Limited >50 m, no aid													
21	Unlimited, with aid	21												
19	Unlimited + aid, slow		19						19					19
18	With aid >50 m										18		18	
16	No aid, limited 8–50 m			16	16					16		16		
15	With aid 8–50 m					15								
14	With aid <8 m+													
12	1 person standby ± aid													
9	1 person hands on ± aid						9							
7	Lying/sitting independently													
4	Positions self in bed													
0	Needs positioning in bed							0						

Fig. 2. Mobility, transfers and balance are shown in separate cases of delirium (Examples 1 and 2) in relation to baseline function (BL). Fluctuation in mobility and balance is observed in both cases. However, in the case where delirium resolves (Example 1), an overall improvement in mobility, to near pre-admission level, is observed. In pre-terminal delirium (Example 2), the nadir of mobility, requiring positioning in bed, total lift for transfers and impaired static standing, presages patient death.

Frailty, Mobility and Age-Related Impairments

There is a consensus that age-related decline occurs across all of the specialized functions that contribute to mobility at the interface of sensory systems, the CNS and neuromotor responses. Disturbance is compounded by specific musculoskeletal system attenuation and contributes to a general decline in balance and mobility in older decades. Both the osteoarthritis and the osteoporosis disease processes are implicated within the frailty cycle, with the combined effect of osteopenia/osteoporosis and sarcopenia implicated in more severe presentations of frailty in older women living in the community [12]. Despite performance diminution with age, not all older adults are frail or ponderous in gait, as Miyazaki Hidekichi, 'the golden bolt' and fastest running centenarian, would attest. Examples aside, the population's propensity for frailty and for more advanced stages of frailty increases with chronological age and is thus significant in subpopulations over 80 years of age.

Performance-based measures and accumulation of deficits more often than not agree on the presence of frailty but may differ in how frailty is identified. What is consistent is the likelihood that early-onset chronic disease is a precursor. Chronic inflammation has been linked to the paradigm of aging and increased adiposity, sarcopenia, reduced muscle strength and decreased mobility as well as elevated mortality risk [13]. These properties are all associated with frailty, particularly in combination. Chronic inflammation, given its antecedent influence, is an attractive and potentially unifying pathophysiological culprit. Mobility is of particular interest, as exercise is also an important preventative intervention against chronic inflammation.

Preliminary evidence from multi-disciplinary and multi-component (strength, endurance, flexibility and balance) exercise programs [14] shows a positive effect on muscle mass and function. Increasing physical fitness and muscle protein anabolism supports interventions even in frail (and obese) individuals. Nutrition, as an important facet of frailty, should be optimized as part of multi-disciplinary treatments in order to realize functional and mobility benefits [15]. The outcomes of such interventions need to be carefully monitored to ensure that a protective effect against falls is achieved while increasing mobility. The quality of the inherent balance training in such programs – along with adherence and participation – are critical factors to consider when 'exercise' is integral to the intervention delivered to older adults.

Frailty, Mobility and Age-Related Impairments: The Frailty Phenotype

Measurement of Frailty and Mobility

The approaches to measurement of frailty have been dealt with earlier in this book. However, in relation to mobility, it is important to highlight the relative merits of these measures. The Fried phenotype, while affording a glimpse of pathophysiological mechanisms implicated in frailty itself (such as sarcopenia), does suffer from the inclusion of mobility items into the derivation of frailty [5]. The loading of mobility in measurement may skew an individual's frailty category, all other things being equal. By contrast, the model of deficit accumulation would appear to be a robust construct of frailty, even when items, such as mobility, are excluded [16].

A comprehensive assessment by a geriatrician is a mandatory starting point for the assessment of frail older adults and provides a framework from which care plans can be managed. The evaluation of the patient should span a biopsychosocial framework. By also incorporating the problems commonly encountered in older patients, the information should then be of clinical utility. Ideally, these data should be directly transferable to frailty assessment to avoid duplication or measurement of items that are not in and of themselves clinically informative or for which collection is considered a burden to the frailest patients. Supplementary information may still be required to refine understanding of a particular function of interest, such as mobility.

The association between frailty, mobility and falls risk – particularly at the upper end of frailty states – is sufficiently clear to mandate an assessment of balance and mobility. The Clinical Frailty Scale [17] is a useful starting point for stratifying (categorizing) presenting patients who may require further evaluation of mobility and balance. Tools can then be selected in line with both the capacity to undertake measures of balance and functional mobility and the outcome performance desired.

For those able to stand and walk, to date, laboratory studies have provided the strongest evidence of the type of clinical balance and mobility assessments that may differentiate frailty in older adults. Gait speed and gait variability, and particularly stride time variability, when walking fast over an electronic walkway compared to a comfortable pace [7] have been consistently linked to more frail older adults, placing them at a higher falls risk. Dual-task protocols that include cognitive distractions while standing more greatly compromise balance control in frail individuals compared to healthier older adults [8]. Thus, measures that include dual tasks and/or the added demand of walking at changing walk speeds or walking as fast as one is able are likely to better differentiate frailty states. Timed rapid gait; the Timed Up and Go test with dual-task components (Cognitive and Manual); and the Functional Gait Assessment, which includes a changing walk speed and specific challenges to walking ability, are more likely to differentiate frail from healthier older adults [18]. As the Functional Gait Assessment correctly predicted 100% of participants who fell within 6 months of testing – a superior outcome to the other tools investigated (Time Up and Go (83%) and Dynamic Gait Index (67%)) – this tool has potential for screening frail older adults who are still ambulant in the community [19]. While further work with frail older adults is indicated, this tool could provide optimal direction for pre-emptive interventions.

Within the acute medical setting (hospital) and/or residential aged care facility, tools that are sensitive to physiological states as well as a range of mobility tasks are required. Given the mobility status of many patients, tools that monitor bed mobility and transfers from bed/chair as well as balance and walking tasks for the more ambulant patient are required so that lower-functioning adults can also be progressively monitored. Several tools stand out in this context, with evidence of reliability and validity for use in the acute ward setting and/or residential care setting, although limited evidence of their ability to predict falls has been reported. The Hierarchical Assessment of Balance and Mobility (HABAM), providing a visual analog interval measure, has demonstrated reliability and validity for use in the acute setting [20]. Unpublished data that were recently reported support earlier research showing that the HABAM is responsive to physiological change, allowing it to be used to track illness and recovery in acute older inpatients [1]. The de Morton Mobility Index is a reliable and valid tool for monitoring functional mobility in a range of settings, with demonstrated responsiveness to a change in functional mobility an older acute medical population [21], although capacity to respond to changing physiological states has not been reported. Another scale for functional mobility, or the Physical Mobility Scale, has been used in residential care facilities to reveal a nonlinear (inverse) association with falls risk among people in these settings [9], but this tool has not been used in the acute ward environment. Each of these measures allows individuals ranging from independent to needing a level of assistance (burden of care) to be monitored during a hospital stay or within home or residential care facilities.

Immobility and Reinforcement of the Frailty Stereotype

What is the conceptual support for mobility intervention in a frail individual? It is known that frailty is not a static paradigm. Transitions to higher levels of frailty are consistently common. Spontaneous improvements are also a reliable observation, but just more infrequent [22]. Thus, the assumption that frailty-related decline is nonrecoverable and therefore that frailty is nonmodifiable is incorrect, except perhaps at the limit of frailty. In cases of improvement, a penumbra of deficit in an individual trait, such as mobility or transfers, may be restored to the point that it becomes an asset. Exploitation of this penumbra with an intervention can be applied to target individual, multiple and disparate functions, with a reduction in aggregate deficits or frailty level. At the outset, the permutations of deficits, even for individuals at the same levels of frailty, are endless. It is understandable, therefore, that multi-disciplinary, multi-faceted and individualized comprehensive geriatric assessment and management are required to target this diversity of deficits, and why this approach works is clear [14, 15]. Nowhere does this apply more clearly than for mobility. It has been established that mobility is an important modifier of prognosis in any given frailty state. Improved mobility, a target for geriatric management, favors stabilization or improvement in frailty [23]. Deficits, alone or in combination, may require a selective evidence base and educationally supported intervention(s). Thus, there is no place for reduced mobility to reinforce the frailty stereotype if both are potentially modifiable. An attitude of treatment opportunity should prevail, and geriatric medicine would indeed be less interesting if this were not the case. The role of physiotherapy is important, enabling functional mobility within a multi-disciplinary management plan, whether in the acute setting or within the community. Interventions may range from determining a safe mode of ambulation to optimizing balance and mobility to reduce falls risk and adverse fall events. Consideration needs to be given to the multiple components of balance and mobility in conjunction with appropriate surface and sensory system challenges as well as dual-task capacity to ensure optimal outcomes [24].

The following questions then arise: What are the levels of frailty at which mobility can be modified? What are the best interventions? Is there a level of frailty at which interventions are no longer effective and therefore cannot be recommended? It is difficult to be prescriptive, but there are at least some principles that should guide the clinician and perhaps organizations. Even at the ceiling of frailty, to the chagrin of otherwise masterful clinicians, life span is a challenge to predict. The frailty limit, regarded as an FI of 2/3 [22], can be appreciated as a terminal condition in waiting. However, the predicament is not governed by the progressive and relentless force of, say, a cancer. Instead, the inability to withstand a stochastic event is predictable only in as much as any random event is, which is not at all. Thus, it remains the case that even in the upper range of frailty, where both modification of the frailty trajectory and mobility improvement are unlikely and life expectancy is limited but unquantifiable, interventions pertaining to mobility must be individualized in the context of the patient's own goals.

Frailty, Mobility and the Dignity of Risk

Advanced levels of frailty are associated with an elevated background risk of adverse events. Falls and injury are predictable consequences. Frequently, the central issue governing the viability of discharge of a frail individual from an acute or subacute setting is mobility impairment. If even after judicious intervention, the risk related to poor mobility remains high, then the outcome is a tussle between autonomy and primum non nocere. This perceived risk may be amplified by social factors such as isolation.

The health professional team may quite reasonably determine, according to the risk of harm to the patient, that alternatives, such as placement for mobility supervision, would be the overriding ethical consideration needed to preserve patient safety. However, autonomy and the dignity of risk take precedence when capacity has been clearly demonstrated. The casualty in clinical practice is frequently the dignity of risk, and the patient's goals in the case of independent living may be subverted. Healthcare teams need to be able to respond to the wishes of the patient after risk evaluation, capacity assessment, optimization and education have taken place, even when that sits uncomfortably with the MDT. If these ethical principles are not embraced, then posterity may bestow the term 'stolen generation' on our demographic of elders who have been placed in high-care residential facilities prematurely. Health professionals have the right to the occasional acts of *outrageous paternalistic hypocrisy* when patient autonomy equates to unbridled calamity. The exercise of professional leverage is called for both in cases of precarious mobility with lacking capacity and when capacity is present but overwhelming risk is absent.

Scope for Intervention in Disorders of Mobility and Frailty

Comprehensive geriatric assessment and MDT evaluation with multi-modal interventions are important in both hospital and community settings [14, 15]. As we have stated, the diversity of problems that patients, even at the same magnitude of frailty, may possess instills the need for individualized management. The contribution of mobility and balance to the frailty state, the suggestion of shared inflammatory pathways and the frequently cited patient goal of (discharge-dependent) mobility make the entities of frailty and mobility amenable to synergistic interventions [25]. Frailty may not only modulate the response to intervention strategies but also dictate their feasibility. In particular, the burden of treatment may be intolerable among the frailest frail [26]. Chapter 12 will explore the theme of 'Frailty and Rehabilitation' in greater depth.

Conclusion

Frailty represents a state of heightened vulnerability. Mobility impairment contributes to the construct of frailty and channels adverse events. While mobility disorder is universal at a high frailty burden, neither mobility nor balance dysfunction is sufficient to fully define frailty. Frailty represents proximity to complex system failure, with higher-order disturbance, such as mobility and balance disturbance, often a consequence. Mobility impairment predicts falls, frequently serving as a black swan event in the life of a frail individual.

Patients with dementia walk too fast for their level of frailty. Conversely, reduced gait speed and gait variability in the absence of dementia are associated with frailty.

Impairment of mobility and balance is a common manifestation of illness and is therefore a sensitive marker of acute disease, putatively also in delirium. Measurement of mobility and balance should therefore be prioritized, and assessment tools such as the de Morton Mobility Index and the HABAM, are being explored, with the sensitivity of the HABAM illustrated in the acute hospital setting. Walking with speed and under dual/multi-task conditions may better differentiate healthier and frail ambulant adults, providing a basis for screening older adults for pre-emptive interventions. Specific mobility and balance interventions have been shown to reduce falls risk, but their acceptability to frail patients remains unproven. The dignity of risk in relation to discharge objectives for a frail, poorly mobile individual frequently divides treatment teams.

Overall, there is no need for reduced mobility to reinforce the frailty stereotype; both are potentially modifiable, and tailored intervention strategies are paramount.

Acknowledgments

We would like to thank Stephanie Yerkovich, chief scientist for the thoracic research unit at The Prince Charles Hospital, for her assistance with manuscript preparation.

References

1 Hubbard RE, Eeles EM, Rockwood MR, Falah N, Ross E, Mitnitski A, Rockwood K: Assessing balance and mobility to track illness and recovery in older inpatients. J Gen Intern Med 2011;26:1471–1478.

2 Fairhall N, Sherrington C, Kurrle SE, Lord SR, Cameron ID: ICF participation restriction is common in frail, community-dwelling older people: an observational cross-sectional study. Physiotherapy 2011;97:26–32.

3 Davis DH, Rockwood MR, Mitnitski AB, Rockwood K: Impairments in mobility and balance in relation to frailty. Arch Gerontol Geriatr 2011;53:79–83.

4 Hubbard RE, Eeles E, Rockwood K: Chapter 105: disorders of mobility and balance; in Brocklehurst's Textbook of Geriatric Medicine and Gerontology, ed 7. Philadelphia, Elsevier, 2010, pp 886–893.

5 Fried LP, Tangen CM, Walston J, Newman AB, Hirsch C, Gottdiener J, Seeman T, Tracy R, Kop WJ, Burke G, McBurnie MA, Cardiovascular Health Study Collaborative Research Group: Frailty in older adults: evidence for a phenotype. J Gerontol A Biol Sci Med Sci 2001;56:M146–M156.

6 van Iersel MB, Verbeek AL, Bloem BR, Munneke M, Esselink RA, Rikkert MG: Frail elderly patients with dementia go too fast. J Neurol Neurosurg Psychiatry 2006;77:874–876.

7 Montero-Odasso M, Muir SW, Hill M, Doherty TJ, Kloseck M, Beauchet O, Speechley M: Gait variability is associated with frailty in community-dwelling older adults. J Gerontol A Biol Sci Med Sci 2011;66:568–576.

8 Kang HG, Coasta MD, Priplata AA, Starobinets OV, Goldberger AL, Peng CK, Kieby DK, Cuplles LA, Lipsitz LA: Frailty and the degradation of complex tasks during a dual task protocol. J Gerontology A Biol Sci Med Sci 2009;64:1304–1311.

9 Barker A, Nitz J, Low Choy N, Haines T: Mobility has a non-linear association with falls, risk among people in residential aged care: an observational study. J Physiother 2012;58:117–125.

10 Slaughter SE, Estabrooks CA: Optimizing the mobility of residents with dementia: a pilot study promoting healthcare aide uptake of a simple mobility innovation in diverse nursing home settings. BMC Geriatr 2013;13:110.

11 Eeles EM, White SV, O'Mahony SM, Bayer AJ, Hubbard RE: The impact of frailty and delirium on mortality in older inpatients. Age Ageing 2012;41:412–416.

12 Frisoli A, Chaves PH, Ingham SJ, Fried LP: Severe osteopenia and osteoporosis, sarcopenia and frailty status in community-dwelling older women: results from the Women's Health and Ageing Study (WHAS) II. Bone 2011;48:952–957.

13 Addison O, LaStayo PC, Dibble LE, Marcus RL: Inflammation, ageing and adiposity: implications for physical therapists. J Geriatr Phys Ther 2012;35:86–94.

14 Cameron I, Fairhall N, Langron C, Lockwood K, Monaghan N, Aggar C, Sherrington C, Lord S, Kurrle S: A multifactorial interdisciplinary intervention reduces frailty in older people: randomized trial. BMC Med 2013;11:65.

15 Singh NA, Quine S, Clemson LM, Williams EJ, Williamson DA, Stavrinos TM, Grady JN, Perry TJ, Lloyd BD, Smith EU, Singh MA: Effects of high-intensity progressive resistance training and targeted multidisciplinary treatment of frailty on mortality and nursing home admissions after hip fracture: a randomized controlled trial. J Gerontol A Biol Sci Med Sci. J Am Med Dir Assoc 2012;13:24–30.

16 Searle SD, Mitnitski A, Gahbauer EA, Gill TM, Rockwood K: A standard procedure for creating a frailty index. BMC Geriatr 2008:30:24.

17 Rockwood K, Song X, Macknight C, Bergman H, Hogan DB, McDowel I, Mitnitski A: A global clinical measure of fitness and frailty in elderly people. CMAJ 2005;173:489–495.
18 Shumway-Cook A, Woollacott MH: Chapter 15: clinical management of the patient with a mobility disorder; in: Motor Control: Translating Research Into Clinical Practice. Philadelphia, Lippincott Williams & Wilkins, 2007, pp 390–440.
19 Wrisley DM, Kumar NA: Functional gait assessment: concurrent, discriminative, and predictive validity in community-dwelling older adults. Phys Ther 2010;90:761–773.
20 MacKnight C, Rockwood K: A hierarchical assessment of balance and mobility. Age Ageing 1995;24: 126–130.
21 de Morton NA, Davidson M, Keating JL: Validity, responsiveness and the minimal clinically important difference for the de Morton Mobility Index (DEMMI) in an older acute medical population. BMC Geriatr 2010;10:72.
22 Mitnitski A, Song X, Rockwood K: Trajectories of change over twelve years in the health status of Canadians from late middle age. Exp Gerontol 2012; 47:893–899.
23 Fallah N, Mitnitski A, Searle SD, Gahbauer EA, Gill TM, Rockwood K: Transitions in frailty status in older adults in relation to mobility: a multistate modeling approach employing a deficit count. J Am Geriatr Soc 2011;59:524–529.
24 Nitz JC, Low Choy NL: The efficacy of a balance strategy training circuit for community based elders who have had a fall. Age Ageing 2004;33:52–58.
25 Heyn PC, Johnson KE, Kramer AF: Endurance and strength training outcomes on cognitively impaired and cognitively intact older adults: a meta-analysis. J Nutr Health Aging 2008;12:401–409.
26 Dorresteijn TA, Zijlstra GA, Delbaere K, van Rossum E, Vlaeyen JW, Kempen GI: Evaluating an inhome multicomponent cognitive behavioural programme to manage concerns about falls and associated activity avoidance in frail community-dwelling older people: design of a randomised control trial [NCT01358032]. BMC Health Serv Res 2011;11:228.

Dr. Eamonn Eeles
4th floor administration
Internal Medicine Services, The Prince Charles Hospital
Rode Road, Chermside, Brisbane, QLD 4032 (Australia)
E-Mail Eamonn.Eeles@health.qld.gov.au

Theou O, Rockwood K (eds): Frailty in Aging. Biological, Clinical and Social Implications.
Interdiscipl Top Gerontol Geriatr. Basel, Karger, 2015, vol 41, pp 121–136 (DOI: 10.1159/000381204)

Frailty and Interprofessional Collaboration

Marion C.E. Briggs[a, d] • Janet E. McElhaney[b, c]

[a]Northern Ontario School of Medicine and [b]Health Sciences North and [c]Advanced Medical Research Institute of Canada, Sudbury, and [d]AMS Phoenix Project, Toronto, Ont., Canada

Abstract

This chapter underscores the importance of interprofessional collaboration in the care of frail older patients. Hospital-based care is emphasized because interprofessionalism is difficult in that setting since the setting is constantly changing and since multiple healthcare professionals care for many complex, very ill patients, only some of whom are frail older people. Interprofessionalism is particularly important and challenging in teaching units in the acute care setting, where many health professionals practice and learn together and team membership changes frequently. Learning is enhanced and interprofessionalism can enhance learning by viewing the patient as a key part of the teaching team. While 'best practice' interventions have been identified for frail older adults who are hospitalized, these interventions are not easily implemented in routine hospital care. Three interdependent processes in clinical practice – representation, sense-making, and improvisation – are described, which contribute to an understanding of how practices change when implemented in a way that takes the local context into account and keeps person-centered care as the central consideration.

Frail older adults are defined by their multiple, interacting medical and social problems. A range of skills is often required to meet their many complex needs and offer meaningful care. These skills typically are shared by many team members, where 'team' expertise evolves through the interdependent and collaborative work of multiple, interdependent disciplines. People in these disciplines need to be able to work together to achieve the best effect. Understandably, bringing together people with different points of view can be a challenge. Perhaps more surprisingly, the challenge is often glossed over. One context in which interprofessionalism and care of the frail older person are infrequently discussed in the literature is the acute care environment, and specifically clinical teaching units (CTUs) where learners from many disciplines could be introduced to and learn about interprofessional collaboration. This chapter contributes conversation to that gap. We begin by introducing the CTU of an academic health sciences center and three frail older patients in that unit. This will situate the reader in a particular context that can be kept in mind as we develop the theoretical elements. We then articulate the case for and some key principles of interprofessionalism (a term that we intend to capture interprofessional collaboration in practice [IPC], education [IPE], and research). Next, we discuss a theoretical framework of practice as a foundation for interprofessionalism and draw attention to three interdependent processes that interact as the practices of/in particular communities: (i) the development and use of practical, locally relevant, evidence-informed practice guidelines and policies (representation); (ii) processes of shared sense-making; and (iii) processes through which the moment-by-moment improvisation is enacted as professionals conduct their practice in the constantly changing clinical environment. Compassionate, person-centered, interprofessional collaborative practices emerge in this interdependent web. We argue that this triad of complex processes (representation, sense-making, and improvisation) constitutes the interdependent process of interprofessionalism in theory and in practice, including practice settings that aspire to provide high-quality care for frail older adults.

Introduction to the Clinical Teaching Unit at the University Health Center

The (fictitious) CTU at the university health center described here is a 38-bed inpatient unit in an academic teaching hospital. We will shortly describe three frail older patients who are among many other patients being cared for in the unit. Of the other 35 patients, 9 are over the age of 70 but are not considered frail, and 2 are designated 'Alternate Level of Care' and are awaiting nursing home placement. The remaining 24 patients are adult patients with a variety of acute conditions, such as heart and/or renal failure; acute exacerbation of chronic lung disease; stroke; sepsis; community-acquired pneumonia; and failure to thrive related to health issues linked to homelessness, mental health issues, and/or substance abuse.

There is a medical director for this service; she is the attending physician 1 week out of 10 but always carries administrative responsibility for medicine. Direct medical care is provided by nine attending physicians who rotate every week, a chief resident on the service for 1 year, one senior and two junior residents who rotate every 1–2 months, and four medical students who rotate every 4 weeks. The unit manager is a nurse who is also responsible for two other hospital units where patients on the teaching service may also be cared for. There is a unit-based charge nurse on every shift. Registered nurses, registered practical nurses, and personal support workers work 12-hour shifts, rotating through 2 day shifts and 2 night shifts followed by 4 days off.

Other full-time unit-based staff include unit clerks, a physiotherapist, an occupational therapist, reactivation workers, a dietician, a social worker, and a respiratory therapist. Part-time staff include a pharmacist, a chaplain, and the cleaning staff. Other staff come and go and interact with patients, such as phlebotomists, x-ray technologists, psychologists, medical consultants, porters, security personnel, patient support workers, and volunteers. Visiting hours are unrestricted, and since many of the patients are extremely ill, it is common for visitors to be present around the clock.

Each weekday, the attending physician, residents, medical students, charge nurse, physiotherapist, occupational therapist, dietician and social worker meet for 'bullet rounds'. Each patient is discussed in rapid succession, and team members are expected to note barriers to discharge and to recommend a treatment plan for the day. Plans are recorded by the charge nurse but are often not communicated to the point-of-care nurses, and while the written record of the plan for the day is available at the nursing station, few nurses read it, and even fewer medical or allied staff refer to it. New staff or those who tend to be introverted often remain silent, so their contributions are easily missed. Some feel intimidated by the whole process. The unit environment feels hectic and disorganized, though the numbers of reported incidents of medication errors, falls, and injuries to patients and staff are quite low. The reader is invited to keep this busy and somewhat unpredictable context in mind and to imagine how interprofessionalism might be enacted in this unit in the context of the reader's own experience in the management of frail older patients.

The Case for Interprofessionalism

Contemporary health services increasingly serve patients with multiple, complex chronic illnesses, and they require interteam and interagency coordination [1]. For older adults suffering acute illness or injury requiring hospitalization, *every hour and every staff encounter counts* to achieve the best possible outcomes. In Canada, over 50% of acute care hospital beds are occupied by seniors (persons aged 65 years and older) on any particular day [2]. About one third of older persons admitted to acute care are discharged at a significantly reduced level of functional ability, and most never recover to their previous level of independence [3]. Hospital costs rise because of complications associated with hospital care, at least some of which are avoidable. Patients and their families/caregivers may also experience unnecessary financial and social costs associated with recurrent admissions, loss of independence and diminished quality of life. Frustrating gaps in care in the transitions between care sectors introduce additional risks. These multifaceted, intersecting issues represent solvable problems for which the development of sustainable solutions must be a top priority.

Comprehensive, interprofessional geriatric assessment and management strategies can prevent readmission to the hospital, but challenges related to collaboration across multiple professions in the transition from the emergency department (ED) to inpatient units and subsequent return to the community can lead to functional decline and an increase in hospital length of stay. Prolonged wait times in busy EDs and delays before treatment is activated are common in hospital wards and also increase risk. Interprofessional collaboration is widely thought to be an essential feature of responsive care processes that address the urgent needs of older adults in acute care settings [4]. The complexity of health issues faced by older adults who are admitted to acute care settings is well known and complicated by the fact that less than 50% of all older adults are up to date on preventive health services [5]. In some settings, older adults take an average of 19 medication doses daily and see 5 specialists and 2 primary care physicians in four different locations each year, very little of which is reported on entry to a hospital setting. In the hospital, an older person admitted for a surgical procedure will see 27 different healthcare providers during the hospital stay, and less than half will follow-up with their primary care physician [5]. A face-value argument in favor of a comprehensive, integrated, interprofessional approach to care for frail older adults, including comprehensive geriatric assessment, is justified and has been shown to minimize these risks [6] (see also Chapter 8).

The World Health Organization [4] concluded that research over the last 50 years shows convincing evidence that health services are optimized and health outcomes improved through effective interprofessional collaborative practice. The same report also acknowledged that there is sufficient evidence to draw causal inferences between effective interprofessional education and effective collaboration in practice. At least in developed countries, modern healthcare systems consist of complex and variably integrated systems that deliver care in multiple sectors (e.g. acute care, rehabilitation, primary care, home and community care, and long-term care) and that involve multiple professions and support staff. Unique disciplines and specialty practices within a single profession have grown exponentially. Often, the theory and technical language as well as the professional culture of different professions, and even those of disciplines within a single profession, can be unintelligible across disciplinary borders [7]. This is all the more challenging for frail older adults and their families. Making sense of healthcare services with and for patients is a goal of interprofessionalism that is often unmet.

The complexity of need is often cited to explain why it is so important that we practice collaboratively in healthcare [8, 9]. Both IPE and IPC have an overarching goal of supporting compassionate, person-centered care, a term that we use to point to the importance of including patients and their families as contributing members of the healthcare team and also to the importance of relationships with and between members of the healthcare team. The Canadian Interprofessional Health Collaborative (CIHC) developed a well-known competency framework for collaborative practice (2010). This framework is being widely used internationally as a guide for the development of interprofessional curricula and interprofessional practice standards (fig. 1 [10]).

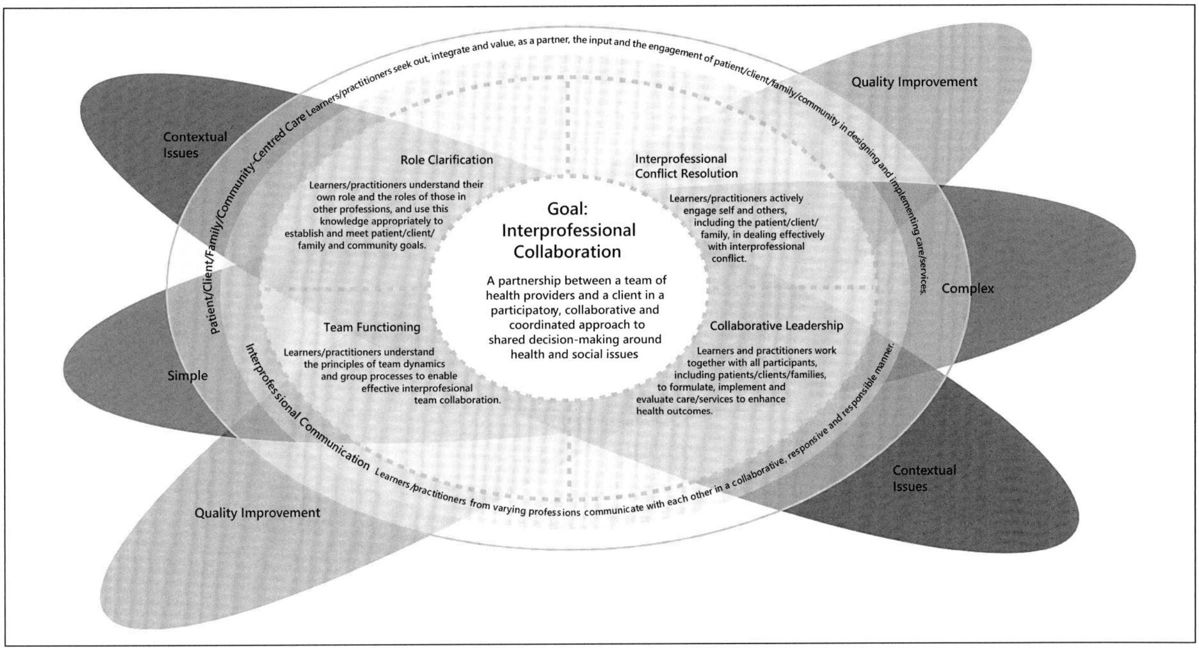

Fig. 1. National interprofessional competency framework.

Key Principles of Interprofessional Collaborative Practice

The 2010 CIHC framework is set against a background of quality improvement and acknowledges the importance of context as well as the continuum of simple to complex circumstances within any given context. The framework then overlays four interprofessional competencies (role clarification, teamwork, collaborative leadership, and interprofessional conflict resolution) on two additional competencies key to all, namely, interprofessional communication and patient-centered care. These six competencies describe the attributes of effective team function and the characteristics required by practitioners to be considered 'interprofessional practice-ready'. Lingard points out that individual and team competence are not linked in a simple, linear way [8]. She argues that (i) competent practitioners do not necessarily come together as a competent team; (ii) a practitioner may effectively collaborate on one team, but not another; and (iii) an incompetent practitioner may unravel one competent team, but not another. In the enactment of these competencies by/between individual practitioners, interprofessionalism becomes a complex 'dance' performed differently in each context and even in multiple ways within a single context as team membership shifts over the course of the day and as the needs of each patient are prioritized considering the needs of all of the patients. Because of this, team principles, practices and strategies for the enactment of interprofessionalism resist 'universal' heuristics and instead emerge in both predictable and unpredictable ways as we work together in real time. We will explore this idea of the emergence of the practices of particular communities in more depth shortly.

As stated, the World Health Organization [4] concluded that evidence links effective IPC, at least in part, to effective IPE. IPE often focuses on the competencies (for example, [10]), which, once mastered, are likely to lead to effective collaboration. Still, it is sometimes easy to lose sight of the patient in this. Bleakley et al. [11] argues that IPE can also be understood as learning 'from, with, and about *patients*', where the patient is the living text. The interprofessional team becomes a resource for learners who have a direct relationship with the patient-as-teacher, which is not mediated by a clinical or academic teacher. Osler's famous quote also speaks to this way of thinking: '... it is a safe rule to have no teaching without a patient for a text, and the best teaching is that taught by the patient himself' [12].

In caring for frail older adults who are hospitalized, the intent and ideology of patients-as-teachers [13] may be challenged by the ability of the patient and his/her family to fully participate. However, engaging with frail older patients and their families as 'text' is a crucial part of creating what Bleakley et al. [1] call a 'knowledge-generating dialogue'. In this way, the patient can literally speak for him/herself so that the intent of collaborative, patient-centered care can be achieved. The text offered by a patient and/or his/her caregivers that are of most interest to each team member might vary, but each potential focus is an important part of the whole person, inclusive of physical, biological, emotional, relational, spiritual, socioeconomic, and environmental aspects of his/her past, current and potential future life story. We suggest that this notion of 'knowledge-generating dialogues' is what crucially distinguishes collaboration from other concepts of team function, such as communication, coordination or cooperation. It is also crucial to understanding the vital role of the patient as part of not only the care team but also the teaching team.

Work by Benner et al. [14] offers three additional principles that are helpful in thinking about (interprofessional) practice. They call for practitioners and teams to develop of a 'sense of salience', citing that since it is impossible to identify every possible contingency in clinical algorithms or care guidelines, practitioners and teams must develop a keen ability to understand what is important. This certainly applies to a particular patient, but it also requires a continuing sensibility to the overall context in which care occurs. The multiple competing demands of the CTU described at the beginning of this chapter, for example, comprise a specific risk to the provision of the right care at the right time for frail older adults, whose urgent need for mobility may need to compete with the equally legitimate needs of acutely ill adults in need of urgent procedural interventions. We suggest that it is in this real-world context of competing legitimate priorities that a deep understanding of 'practice' is critical to the development of a functional approach to interprofessionalism.

The second principle that Benner et al. [14] call for is integrative thinking. Integrative thinking promotes clinical intuition, in which, through continuing conversations, practitioners draw on propositional and situational knowledge, professional judgment, skilled know-how, and ethical comportment to anticipate the outcome of particular interventions. Doctors do not prescribe analgesics, and nurses do not give these drugs just to see what will happen; they anticipate that the particular pain that a patient is experiencing will be significantly less within a given time, and if it is not, adjustments to dose

Table 1. Key competencies/characteristics of interprofessionalism

Key competencies/aptitudes of interprofessionalism	
CIHC interprofessional competencies [10]	Benner et al. [14]
Patient/client/family/community-centered care	A sense of salience
Interprofessional communication	Clinical imagination
Role clarification	Moral imagination
Interprofessional conflict resolution	
Team functioning	
Collaborative leadership	

and/or frequency or an alternate view of the patient's condition can be considered. Effective interprofessional practices build clinical intuition, and team members rely on each other to develop a robust, integrated approach to the generation of relevant clinical knowledge, not only for a particular patient but also for the context in which they are providing care for multiple patients. Integrative thinking is part of what generates the habits and routines of a team and contributes to the development of improvisational skills that are needed among team members to manage multiple emerging demands that cannot be fully predicted. This emergent property of healthcare is described by Bleakley [1] as one in which '... stability is replaced by... a permanent state of fluidity, resulting in a complex context that carries with it high levels of uncertainty'. Emerging population demographics and the increasing challenge of hospitalized frail older adults create some of the most complex challenges in healthcare environments that are, themselves, inherently complex. Effective and fluid collaboration among team members is essential.

Finally, Benner et al. call for the development of moral imagination, by which they mean the ability to quickly form effective relationships and to act with compassion, whether imparting news of a difficult diagnosis, talking about options of care, inserting an intravenous catheter, changing ventilator tubing, doing an assessment, or interacting with team members. Most healthcare encounters are brief; many are less than a minute, and this is also true of many encounters between healthcare providers on a team. Developing moral imagination invites a different way to conceive of the importance of these encounters, however brief or technical they might be. Table 1 summarizes the six CIHC competencies and adds the three additional aptitudes suggested by Benner et al.

Interprofessional Collaboration Reconsidered

Interprofessional collaboration is thought to be a phenomenon that is context specific, meaning that there is no single right way [15]; is responsive, evolving and emergent [16]; and involves continuous interaction and interdependence [17]. These characteristics are consistent with ideas put forward by practice and organizational theorists such as Nicolini [18], Sandberg and Tsoukas [19], and Bourdieu [20]; social theorists such as Flyvbjerg et al. [21]; and medical education and social theorists such as Hodges and Lingard [8]. Not uncommonly, healthcare providers are taught and come to believe that they act independently and have the ability to make unencumbered decisions through independent cognitive and interpretive processes. Moreover, even though there is a broad understanding that 'best and evidence-informed practice' must be modified to suit individual circumstances, continued use of the 'knowledge translation' metaphor in healthcare suggests that we cling to the hope of stability and standardization that make it is possible to literally translate best practice guidelines into our daily practice. Similarly, standard interprofessional team development typically focuses on gaining agreement on the team's mission, vision, values and goals, understanding of roles and the scopes of practice of each discipline (which increases understanding of each discipline's competencies and contributions but may also strengthen professional boundaries and reduce collaboration), generating agreement about the rules of engagement and carefully defining team processes. Collectively, these agreements are often known as 'team charters' and align with a 'will-to-stability' that may frustrate the 'will-to-adaptability' required to accommodate the frequently changing circumstances of the clinical environment [1]. Too often, as we hope that the reader has now noticed, the focus on compassionate and person-centered care has gone missing!

The conditions under which team members must act, particularly in acute care CTUs, change faster than it takes particular ways of acting to become habitual or routine. Acute care contexts in particular are plagued with frequent changes in practice occasioned by new practice guidelines, new equipment, or new policy. Often, the sense is that one change is barely implemented before the next one comes along. Or the next patient comes along. Or one of the patients whom we are responsible for takes an unexpected turn. Or a staff member calls in sick and is replaced by someone not familiar with the caseload or the service. Or a relationship that is tenuous at best erupts into overt hostility. Or a patient falls and is injured. Or an in-service education session takes six staff off the floor. Or there is a shift change. The imagined stability of formal, well-defined team processes cannot take into account the degree to which the practices of any given community face frequent shifts in priorities as the moment-by-moment clinical circumstances emerge in ways that are not always predictable. Specific practices in a care community (such as the CTU that we described) arise and become articulated through algorithms and best practice guidelines but are enacted through processes in which team members (including patients) together make sense about what is needed and what is possible and through processes in which team members (including patients) then negotiate action on clinical decisions within the complex and changes clinical circumstances they encounter [22]. We argue that algorithms and guidelines give us guidance about what to do, but making sense of the way in which guidelines apply in particular circumstances and how we work together to enact them is a critical element of collaborative practice and should be given equal weight when thinking about our practices. Figure 2 shows person-centered care in the intersection between all three process domains.

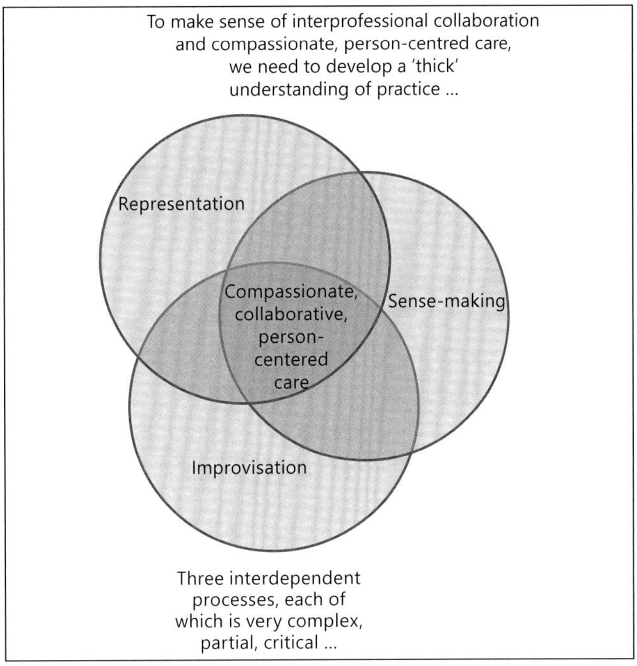

Fig. 2. The three interrelated processes of practice.

Three Interdependent Processes of Practice

Practitioners simultaneously act in all three of the process domains described above. We do not mean to imply a specific starting point or sequence, but suggest that actions in all three domains are likely to occur simultaneously and iteratively. We do mean to show how different ways of knowing and acting influence our collective and individual practices. This will help us to understand teamwork and interprofessionalism as emergent contextual actions undertaken by practitioners and patients, and not as a stable set of idealized principles. Practice theorist Theodore Schatzki [23] argues that practices provide the 'conditions of intelligibility' for action; that is, the practices of particular communities [24] explain why certain actions make sense and others do not. These conditions define, to some extent, what can and cannot be seen, said or done and explain why, for example, practices can be different between different units in one hospital and between similar services in one hospital compared to another, even though similar services rely on the same 'best practice guidelines' and organizational policies. Practices – what Bourdieu [20] calls 'habitus', or the way in which people in particular contexts tend to act – largely arise from the ongoing interactions between the members of a particular community of practice, and much less from the correct translation of science, the blind enactment of policies, or the perfect execution of strategic plans or professional competencies designed to generate specific outcomes [25]. We do not mean to imply that guidelines, policies and competencies are unimportant or that they do not influence practices. It is just that approaches to changing practice must also take into account the importance of the processes of sense-making among interdependent people as they negotiate and improvise their work. An important reason for taking this more complex view is that we do not generally experience 'perfect' patients, with the one problem for which these policies, competencies, or best practices were designed.

Figure 2 shows the three domains of practice that we have been discussing. Practices, including interprofessional practices, are a thoroughly social and emergent phenomenon constituted by interdependent and iterative processes of representation (such as policies and practice guidelines), sense-making (through negotiation and reflective and reflexive practices), and improvisation (deciding how to act in the circumstances at the point and in the moments of care) [22]. In the following sections, we briefly outline some elements that are likely to influence practice in each of these process domains. Compassionate, person-centered care is the central focus in this scheme. We use the term 'person-centered care' (as opposed to 'patient-centered care') to reflect care processes and decision-making that include a broad concern for inclusion of and respectful, knowledge-generating relationships with patients and families and between staff (including physicians).

Processes of Representation

An outcome of the dominance of modern scientific tradition is the search for more precise, more 'accurate' descriptions ('representations') thought to come closer and closer to a final 'truth', or the pre-given essence of a thing (see fig. 3). This approach values objectivism and hypothesis-driven deductive scientific methods. Findings are represented in documents such as best practice guidelines, clinical algorithms and practice guidelines, policies, professional regulatory guidelines, and even strategic planning; particularly in healthcare, reliance on these methods has also resulted in the development of 'implementation science' [26], such as Roger's *Diffusion of Innovation* [27]. Clinically, this way of thinking includes the use of various technically based forms of assessment, including metrics like lab values and imaging, which represent the state of health of an organ or physiologic system. Aristotle referred to this way of thinking as 'episteme', from which the modern term 'epistemology' (scientific knowledge) is derived [21]. When interprofessional teams are described in documents in terms of such aspects as roles and responsibilities, the scope of practice, strategic plans, goals and objectives, policies and procedures, and rules of engagement, this representation of 'teamness' reflects a will-to-stability and predictability [1] and ignores the complex and changing contexts in which team members must practice. Even so, these clinical and team representations in practice are helpful in terms of orienting thought and activity, establishing a sense of shared purpose and effort, and postulating ideals that teams might strive toward. What a document cannot do is make sense of the contingent and unique circumstances in which they are to be applied or reform itself in response to the generation of new practice-based knowledge [28].

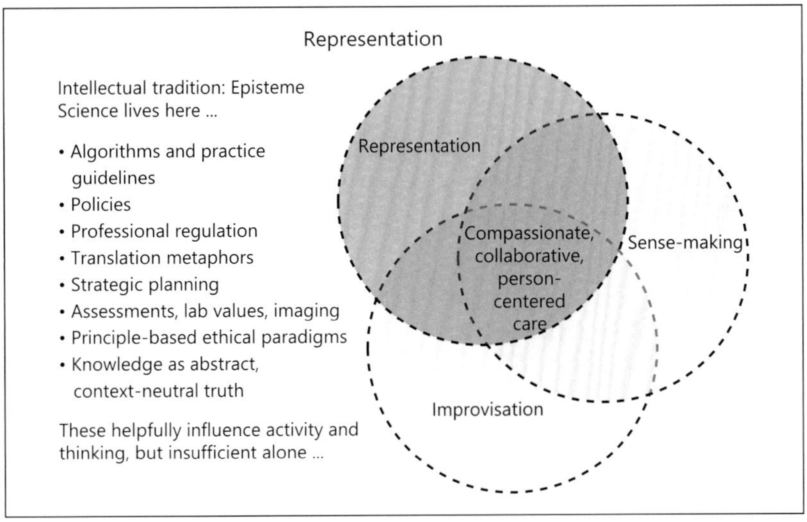

Fig. 3. Processes of representation.

Processes of Sense-Making

People, and not guidelines, make sense of the representations of practice in both clinical and team function contexts (see fig. 4). The importance of this self-evident truth is easily dismissed even though guidelines and other representations of practice are developed from questions that arise in practice. Stacey [25] draws attention to the fact that practice and theory are not dichotomous – that is, separate entities wherein in one moment, we practice, and in another, we theorize – but rather are paradoxically two aspects of the same phenomenon in which both are always at play. This makes sense when we think about the difference between a novice and an experienced practitioner or between a seasoned team and one recently formed to provide a new service. The novice practitioner or new team might rely more heavily on representations initially but will soon begin to reform theory based on experience. In the team context, interprofessional collaboration is supported by making explicit the processes of understanding the application of guidelines or policies in the context of specific patients or circumstances.

The processes involved in sense-making include activities such as reflective and reflexive practices, discussing and coming to agreement on shared goals, collaborative decision-making, discernment of the salient features of complex circumstances, use of multiple ways of thinking, and the development of clinical and moral imagination [14, 22]. A feature that distinguishes collaboration from other processes, such as communication, cooperation or coordination, is the idea of knowledge-generating dialogues [1] between team members, including patients and families. Communication transmits information, cooperation is a relational stance for mutual benefit, and coordination is a sequencing strategy. Collaboration consists of conversation in which new knowledge that did not previously exist is (or could be) generated and informs further deliberation

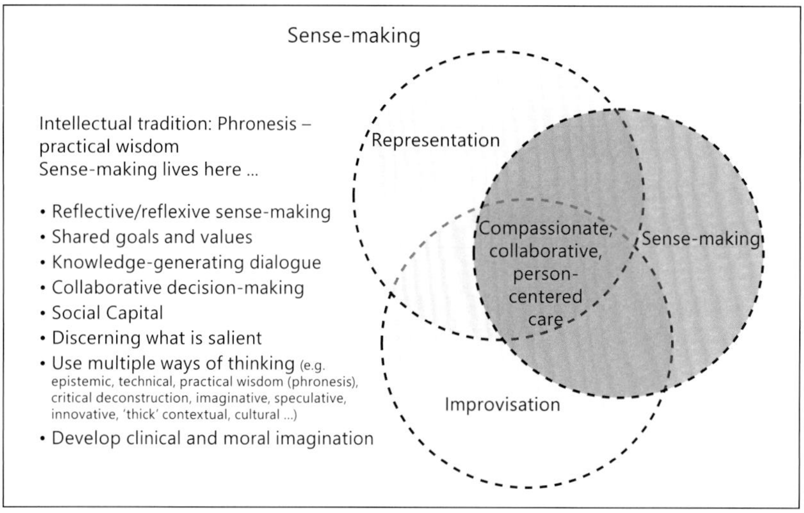

Fig. 4. Processes of sense-making.

and/or action in ways that no one person would have come to on his/her own. With this understanding of collaboration, we see that not every clinical circumstance or team function need be collaborative. It is perfectly appropriate at times to simply communicate or coordinate, and most of the time, tacit agreements around cooperation are part of the social contract of our practices. A face-value argument can be made, stating that the work of true collaboration – or of knowledge-generating conversations – would not be productive if applied in every situation. Complex situations in which diagnosis and treatment options are not at all clear or in which managing challenging interpersonal dynamics within teams or between providers and patients is difficult to get through would benefit from a collaborative approach. Much of what we call interprofessional collaborative practice is not true collaboration and does not need to be. The fact that collaboration is not needed in all circumstances and that it is not generally understood as knowledge-generating dialogues may contribute to the frequently expressed sentiment that it is difficult to find model collaborative practice settings where students can experience and learn to apply what they have learned about IPC in educational settings.

The intellectual tradition that Aristotle most closely associated with sense-making is 'phronesis' [21]. Aristotle thought that phronesis (practical wisdom) was the most important of the intellectual traditions, and unlike for episteme (which translates to the modern term 'epistemology') or techne (which translates to the modern terms 'technique' and 'technology'), there is no modern translation of the word. However, it is an intuitive truth that all healthcare practitioners rely on practical wisdom more and more as they gain experience that re-forms their theory. It is the complex, interacting needs of frail older patients in the hospital that are forcing us to re-think how models of care and care plans can be used to help practitioners gain experience in dealing with those issues, which goes beyond best or evidence-informed practice.

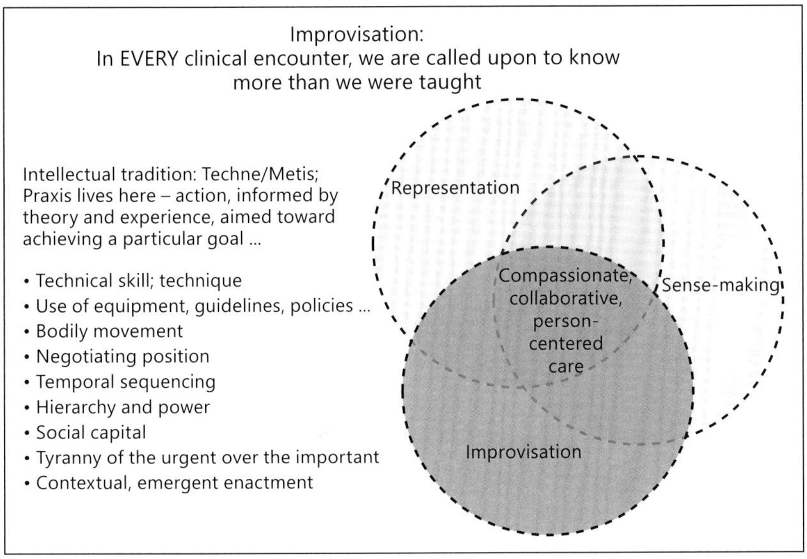

Fig. 5. Processes of improvisation.

Processes of Improvisation

Representation processes expose what we believe that we ought to do in a general and acontextual sense. Processes of Sense-making occur between people who are deeply engaged in a given practice to understand what the next step is, given the unique circumstances in the particular situation in which they must act. Processes of improvisation are those of application (see fig. 5). This is where the rubber hits the road: where best practice has been carefully considered in light of contingent circumstances that we face and where we bring to bear our experience, knowledge (tacit and explicit) and skills and, finally, take the next step. We take action, action that, in every clinical encounter and every team encounter, calls on us to know more than we were taught and that we have never before experienced in quite the same way. There is, of course, a great deal more carryover of thinking and action compared to what might be new. Thus, there is no intent to imply that our actions are random, entirely invented, or without the strong foundation of knowledge, skills, and attitudes. However, improvisation is always needed: what priorities are most important, what equipment is or is not available, what state of mind the patient is in, whether other practitioners have completed tasks that are prerequisite to the action that you must take. We almost always act with others, and this calls on us to negotiate differences in focus, professional and personal values, professional identity and power potential; that is, to attend to our own sense of what needs to happen, balanced with ethical considerations, professional regulation, and policies and guidelines. Processes of improvisation recognize the interdependence of these and other factors that influence what decisions and action are available for us and then help to decide what the next action to follow might be.

Aristotle's final two intellectual traditions, techne and metis, influence improvisation most. 'Techne' has been translated to our modern notions of technique and technology, or psychomotor skills and aptitudes. 'Metis' refers to something like practical wisdom but additionally refers to a kind of 'cunning', such as a sense of when to perform an action that, in most circumstances, would not be consistent with 'best practice'. A practitioner might, for example, rely on metis to start or stop a particular treatment when he/she is still unable to quite say why he/she is making that decision, or the 'gut feel' decision that all seasoned practitioners make that they sometimes find difficult to explain to students. This is particularly relevant to managing end-stage disease in frail older people, when what 'ought' to happen may be difficult to say with any certainty.

We suggest that these three interdependent process domains are what we are doing when we work together in a particular practice community: that is, interprofessional collaboration in a particular practice setting. In the concluding section of this chapter, we will return to reflect further on the context that we described at the beginning, namely, a CTU in the acute care setting, and to explore the notion of whether or not there is a single best practice for the interprofessional management of frail older adults in this setting.

Summary

Over the last two decades, there has been growing evidence for specific 'elder-friendly' interventions and models of care in single care locations within a hospital, such as the ED [29, 30] and inpatient settings [31–33]. These studies have demonstrated both economic and social benefits of interprofessional care, including reductions in length of stay, readmissions and inappropriate resource utilization. Even though many successful interventions have been identified as best practice and have good evidence to support their development and broad implementation [34], effective interventions are not always easily transferred from clinical studies and implemented in routine hospital care [35]. We argue that the 'representation' of practice established in these studies is only the first step. Locally relevant modifications must be made in each care setting through local processes of sense-making and 'improvisation' and then re-presented as new theory derived from practice wisdom. Many traditional models of implementation of care plans (typically within the nursing discipline) or geriatric consultation services (typically physician-driven) may fail to engage the care team in the collaboration (knowledge-generating dialogues) required for truly person-centered care. Particularly in a setting with many competing demands and priorities, such as a CTU, we speculate that practices are especially challenging to articulate and change. The 'reciprocal mentorship' implied by the notion of collaboration as knowledge-generating dialogues invites interprofessionalism into the learning and practice environment in its broadest sense. Our individual and collective experience contributes to the evidence informing *our* best practice as that ideal applies to THIS patient in THESE particular circumstances; there is no universal magic bullet. If we genuinely understand and accept that there is no magic bullet, we would need to completely rethink how practices change and to take very seriously how the three interdependent processes of practice interact every day through every encounter to build our theory/practice paradigms. We suggest that multiple models of care intersecting in complementary ways are needed to effectively address the complex practice and education issues, including competing priorities that get in the way of providing appropriately responsive care for management of the urgent needs of frail older adults. The question of whether it is best to manage hospitalized frail older adults as a cohort population is complex and will be even more so as older adults comprise a larger and larger proportion of the hospitalized population. Will it even be possible to consider older adults as a cohort going forward? Will there be sufficient numbers of geriatricians and other healthcare personnel skilled and interested in the management of frail older adults, or will we need everyone to understand and manage this population, no matter where they are located? Integrating specialized geriatrics services within general populations seems to be a more likely strategy and will require the deep understanding of and engagement with the integrated processes of practices that we have proposed.

Acknowledgments

MCEB acknowledges the support of the 'AMS Phoenix Project: A Call to Caring' in this work.

References

1 Bleakley A: Working in 'teams' in an era of 'liquid' healthcare: what is the use of theory? J Interprof Care 2013;27:18–26.
2 CIHI Discharge Abstract Database – http://www.cihi.ca/CIHI?ext?portal/internet/EN/Quick_Stats/quick+stats/quick_stats_main?xQSType=InteractiveData&pageNumber=2&resultCount=10&filterTypeBy=2&filterTopicBy=undefined&autorefresh=1# (Accessed July 26, 2011).
3 Covinsky KE, Eng C, Lui LY, et al: The last 2 years of life: functional trajectories of frail older people. J Am Geriatr Soc 2003;51:492–498.
4 World Health Organization: Framework for action on interprofessional education and collaborative practice. 2010. http://www.who.int/hrh/resources/framework_action/en/ (accessed May 21, 2014).
5 Institute of Medicine: Best Care at Lower Cost: The Path to Continuously Learning Health Care in America. Washington, DC, The National Academies Press, 2013.
6 Caplan GA, Williams AJ, Daly B, et al: A randomized, controlled trial of comprehensive geriatric assessment and multidisciplinary intervention after discharge of elderly from the emergency department–the DEED II study. J Am Geriatr Soc 2004;52:1417–1423.
7 Hall P: Interprofessional teamwork: professional cultures as barriers. J Interprof Care 2005;(suppl 1): 188–196.
8 Hodges BD, Lingard L: The Question of Competence: Reconsidering Medical Education in the 21st Century. Ithaca, NY, Cornell University Press, 2012.
9 Thistlewaite J: Values-Based Interprofessional Collaborative Practice: Working Together in Health Care. Cambridge, Cambridge University Press, 2012.
10 Canadian Interprofessional Health Collaborative (CIHC): 2010. https://www.cihc.ca/resources/publications 9/23/20 (accessed December 12, 2012).
11 Bleakley A, Bligh J, Browne J: Medical Education for the Future: Identify, Power and Location. New York, Springer, 2011.

12 Osler W: The Hospital as a College. Aeguanimatus and Other Addresses Chapter XVI. London, HK Lewis, 1905.
13 Spencer J, Godolphin W, Karpenko N, et al: Can Patients Be Teachers? Involving Patients and Service Users in Healthcare Professional Education. London, The Health Foundation, 2011.
14 Benner P, Suthpen M, Leonard V, et al: Educating Nurses: A Call for Radical Transformation. San Francisco, CA, Jossey-Bass, 2010.
15 Health Canada: Enhancing interdisciplinary collaboration in primary health care: a change process to support collaborative practice. 2006. http://www.apps.hc-sc.gc.ca/hcs-sss/phctf-fassp.nsf/lkAttachments/7C63B73389EA76D88525728F00667E7A/$File/05E_SUM_EnhanceCollab.pdf (accessed June, 2007).
16 Lahey W, Currie R: Regulatory and medico-legal barriers to interprofessional practice. J Interprof Care 2005;19(suppl 1):197–223.
17 D'Amour D, Iabdasab I: Interprofessional Education for Collaborative Patient-Centred Practice: An Evolving Framework. Chapter 10. Ottawa, Canada, Queen's Printer, 2004.
18 Nicolini D: Practice Theory, Work & Organization: An Inroduction. Oxford, Oxford University Press, 2013.
19 Sandberg J, Tsoukas H: Grasping the logic of practice: theorizing through practical rationality. Acad Manage Rev 2011;36:338–360.
20 Bourdieu P: Outline of a Theory of Practice. Nice R (trans). Cambridge, Cambridge University Press, 1977.
21 Flyvbjerg B, Landman T, Schran S: Real Social Science: Applied Phronesis. Cambridge, Cambridge University Press, 2013.
22 Briggs MCE: Complexity and the Practices of Communities in Health Care: Implications for an Internal Practice Consultant; thesis, School of Business, University of Hertfordshire, Hatfield, UK, 2012, p 195.
23 Schatzki TR: The sites of organizations. Organizational Studies 2005;26:465–484.
24 Gherardi S: Community of practice or practices of a community; in Armstrong S, Fukami C (eds): Handbook of Management Learning, Education, and Development. London, Sage, 2009.
25 Stacey RD: Complexity and Organizational Reality: Uncertainty and the Need to Rethink Management After the Collapse of Investment Capitalism, ed 2. London, Routledge, 2010.
26 Stacey RD: Strategic Management and Organizational Dynamics: The Challenge of Complexity, ed 5. Essex, Prentice Hall, 2007.
27 Rogers JC, Holm MB, Beach S, et al: Concordance of four methods of disability assessment using performance in the home as the criterion method. Arthritis Rheum 2003;49:640–647.
28 Gabbay J, Le May A: Practice-Based Evidence for Healthcare: Clinical Mindlines. New York, Routledge, 2011.
29 McCusker J, Cole M, Dendukuri N, et al: Delirium in older medical inpatients and subsequent cognitive and functional status: a prospective study. CMAJ 2001;165:575–583.
30 Mion LC, Palmer RM, Meldon SW, et al: Case finding and referral model for emergency department elders: a randomized clinical trial. Ann Emerg Med 2003;41:57–68.
31 Inouye SK, Bogardus ST Jr, Baker DI, et al: The Hospital Elder Life Program: a model of care to prevent cognitive and functional decline in older hospitalized patients. Hospital Elder Life Program. J Am Geriatr Soc 2000;48:1697–1706.
32 Landefeld CS, Palmer RM, Kresevic DM, et al: A randomized trial of care in a hospital medical unit especially designed to improve the functional outcomes of acutely ill older patients. N Engl J Med 1995;332: 1338–1344.
33 Naylor MD, Brooten D, Campbell R, et al: Comprehensive discharge planning and home follow-up of hospitalized elders: a randomized clinical trial. JAMA 1999;281:613–620.
34 Rockwood K: Capacity, population aging and professionalism. CMAJ 2006;174:1689, 1691.
35 Reuben DB: Making hospitals better places for sick older persons. J Am Geriatr Soc 2000;48:1728–1729.

Dr. Marion C.E. Briggs
Northern Ontario School of Medicine
935 Ramsay Lake Road, Rm 233 HSERC
Sudbury, ON P3E 2C6 (Canada)
E-Mail mbriggs@nosm.ca

Theou O, Rockwood K (eds): Frailty in Aging. Biological, Clinical and Social Implications.
Interdiscipl Top Gerontol Geriatr. Basel, Karger, 2015, vol 41, pp 137–150 (DOI: 10.1159/000381229)

Frailty and Rehabilitation

Ian D. Cameron[a] · Susan E. Kurrle[b]

[a]John Walsh Centre for Rehabilitation Research, Sydney Medical School Northern, The University of Sydney, Kolling Institute, Royal North Shore Hospital, St Leonards, N.S.W., and [b]Division of Rehabilitation and Aged Care, Hornsby Ku-ring-gai Health Service, Hornsby, N.S.W., Australia

Abstract

Rehabilitation approaches to frailty are in the early stages of development. Frailty also shows promise as a prognostic indicator for rehabilitation programs, similar to its application in other areas of medicine. However, care should be taken not to exclude frail older people from rehabilitation, as has been the case at some centers for people with cognitive impairment or very severe disability. There are clear theoretical reasons to expect that a rehabilitation approach will be effective. Some experimental data are also available suggesting that rehabilitation is effective in frail and pre-frail older people. The principles of a frailty intervention program that have been demonstrated to be clinically and economically effective are as follows: first, frailty can be mitigated; second, support needs are individually addressed; third, the interventions aim to improve physical, cognitive and social functioning; fourth, support has to be delivered over a long time period; and finally, systems must facilitate consistent management. Most frail older people are encouraged and supported to adhere to their intervention plan. It is important to recognize the needs of families and/or carers and to engage with them.

Older people with disabilities are frequent participants in rehabilitation programs [1], and rehabilitation has been shown to be effective for older people with high-prevalence diseases or injuries [2, 3]. Most older people participating in rehabilitation programs fit the definitions of frailty [4]. Depending on the conceptualization of frailty, it might be a temporary or permanent state. If frailty is conceptualized as a temporary state, then rehabilitation is likely to facilitate its resolution.

The objectives of this chapter are to describe approaches to rehabilitation in frail older people, to examine frailty as a mediating factor in establishing the rehabilitation potential of older people, and to illustrate the components of a frailty rehabilitation program that have been shown to be effective.

Defining Rehabilitation

Rehabilitation programs aim to restore the functional capacities of disabled individuals and to prevent further disability [5]. The major goal of rehabilitation programs for older people is to assist them with managing personal activities of daily living without the assistance of another person. If this is not possible, then their goal is to minimize the need for external assistance through the use of adaptive techniques and equipment. It is important for health care professionals who work with older people to be able to recognize both their need for rehabilitation and their potential to benefit from such a program.

Rehabilitation services can be provided in a wide range of settings, depending on the patient needs and service availability. These settings include traditional inpatient rehabilitation wards and outpatient clinics, and rehabilitation is increasingly being provided in other settings, such as the home, acute hospital wards and high-dependency units, to assist in preventing functional decline [6]. The provision of rehabilitation services requires an interdisciplinary approach utilizing a wide range of health care professionals (including nursing, medical, physiotherapy, occupational therapy, speech pathology, social work, and psychology professionals) working together with the patient and his or her family.

The International Classification of Functioning, Disability and Health (ICF) has provided a conceptual framework for rehabilitation that is used extensively in the provision of rehabilitation services and can be used to define goals and targets for interventions [5].

Most older people with a recent significant disability or deterioration in a pattern of stable disability have the potential to benefit from rehabilitation. Chronological age *per se* should not be a factor in determining participation in a rehabilitation program. The major considerations are the ability to benefit from rehabilitation and the ability to cooperate with therapy. The prime determinants are the severity of the presenting disability and the extent of any coexisting condition, such as frailty, that may influence the patient's ability to participate in a rehabilitation program.

Frailty in the Context of Rehabilitation

As described elsewhere in this book, frailty can be conceptualized in a number of ways. Broadly, there are phenotypic and accumulated deficit models [7]. Frailty in the context of rehabilitation is mentioned in the ICF and World Report on Disability (page 100 and page 304 of the glossary) [8], but it is not examined in detail. This lack of detail is not unexpected because it is a recently conceptualized condition.

Rehabilitation is currently provided to frail older people with established disabilities. However, rehabilitation can theoretically be appropriate for older people who may not be considered disabled but who are 'pre-frail', with the goal of improving body function or the ability to perform higher-intensity functional activities – for example, activities requiring more than 3–5 metabolic equivalents of task.

A potentially important question is whether there is a steeper rate of decline in functioning, either acutely or chronically, in frail individuals. This decline could be important because of sub-clinical changes due to homeostatic instability. There is also a known nonlinear relationship of functional performance and disability, defined as restrictions in daily activities, such as mobility [9]. Therefore, frail people near the disability threshold for basic daily self care and domestic activities are vulnerable to decline.

Rehabilitation in frailty can be seen as broadly improvements in functioning, as well as in areas specifically relevant to each individual older person. According to this conceptualization, rehabilitation is potentially applicable for both older people with a disability associated with frailty and for older people with a lesser degree of frailty associated with sub-clinical functional limitations. For example, a mildly frail or pre-frail (using a phenotypic frailty definition) older person may not report a disability but may be unable to achieve sufficient mobility to walk up three flights of stairs. If the aim of the older person is to be able to walk to this extent to access a friend's home, this could be a goal for a rehabilitation program.

Rehabilitation is generally seen as goal-oriented and time-limited. Goals can relate to 'deficits', such as impairments in mobility or the ability to bathe, low mood, or aspects of the frailty phenotype, such as feelings of exhaustion or a low activity level. The approach of rehabilitation is to identify goals (i.e. deficits) that the older person prioritizes so that he or she will be more likely to be adherent with the suggested interventions.

Attempts have been made to categorize rehabilitation approaches, and the World Health Organization is working on a classification of health interventions that will include components of rehabilitation [10]. However, this classification has not been finalized, and no draft versions are currently available.

Because of the increasing use of the ICF in health care and planning associated with health care, the suggested approach is to identify goals relevant to older people with varying degrees of frailty that are consistent with the categorizations of the ICF.

Older people may also have health conditions or limitations (that could be functional, psychological or social) of which they are unaware. Therefore, an additional approach is to perform a comprehensive geriatric assessment (CGA). CGA 'is a process that determines an older person's medical, psychosocial, functional, and environmental resources and problems, and it creates an overall plan for treatment and follow-up' [11].

CGA is often a component of rehabilitation programs involving older people. It has been scientifically validated and has been shown to be effective if carefully applied and followed up in suitable groups of older people [12]. It also can be used to guide care planning and to generate a frailty index.

Frailty and Potential Rehabilitation Approaches

Frailty is generally seen as a progressive state that is associated with unfavorable outcomes, including disability, the requirement for residential care, and death. Despite these associations, the ability to influence changes in the frailty state is of importance to older people.

However, it is not at all clear whether frailty is a static state once it has developed. Depending on the conceptualization of frailty, there are components that can change, either spontaneously through the resolution of illness or injury or through an intervention that might be related to health care or other factors, for example, family support. Therefore, rehabilitation approaches to frailty, pre-frailty and frailty at early stages should be feasible.

Frailty as a 'Risk Factor' in Rehabilitation Programs

Frailty is being reported as a risk factor for poorer outcome in a range of health conditions and with reference to specific treatments, such as cardiac surgery, colorectal surgery [13] and chemotherapy [14]. There have been increasing reports of frailty as a negative prognostic factor for older people participating in rehabilitation programs. This finding has been reported with reference to hip fractures and more broadly with reference to geriatric rehabilitation [4, 15, 16].

These reported associations are not surprising because frailty is highly correlated with disability, as measured at the commencement of the rehabilitation program or prior to the onset of the health condition or injury that led to the requirement for rehabilitation. More severe disability is well known to be a negative prognostic factor for greater improvement in functioning in rehabilitation programs. In this context, the use of frailty as a prognostic factor may be largely acting as a surrogate for known predictors of outcome in these programs.

Rehabilitating Frailty: Broader Empirical Research

Programs to assist older people to live independently and to recover as fully as possible after injury and illness have been described over the last half-century. These programs have had variable effectiveness, and there are many examples of such effective programs [17, 18].

Whether these programs can be considered to be approaching frailty from a rehabilitation perspective is open to discussion. A review of these programs [19] has highlighted that none of them have explicitly measured the frailty of included participants using an accepted definition.

Intervention in Pre-Frailty

To the best of our knowledge, the only study that has explicitly enrolled pre-frail older people was that of Drey and colleagues, who have used frailty criteria to target an exercise program to these individuals. They have defined pre-frailty as the presence of one or two of the five Cardiovascular Health Study criteria and have shown that exercise has the potential to improve functional ability in these pre-frail older people [20].

The Frailty Intervention Trial (FIT) approach, which has been used in the treatment of frailty, has now been extended to pre-frailty. A randomized trial of the treatment of pre-frailty (using the Cardiovascular Health Study criteria) has been conducted using a multifactorial interdisciplinary intervention, incorporating comprehensive geriatric rehabilitation [21]. The initial impressions of this trial are that the goals of pre-frail older people are different than those of frail older people because they experience less disability. In addition, pre-frail older people have a substantially greater capacity for physical activity, which translates into more strenuous exercise programs with higher-level goals with reference to community participation.

The Frailty Intervention Trial Program

The FIT program is an interdisciplinary, multifactorial intervention developed to ameliorate frailty. It was a component of a larger research program investigating 'transitions' in older people. Transitions were conceptualized as changes in the lives of older people that could be related to health, disability, personal factors (for example, the death of a spouse) or environmental factors (such as moving to another accommodation).

Frailty in the FIT program was identified as a state of transition between independence and disability. Frailty has a complex relationship with health conditions and personal and environmental factors [5]. Health professionals working in rehabilitation services assist older people to live as independently as possible; thus, this transitional state was considered to be a potential target for intervention.

The FIT program research group was interdisciplinary, involving medicine (geriatrics and rehabilitation), nursing, physiotherapy, psychology and health economics professionals. Based on this background, the FIT-preferred intervention involved the utilization of a range of approaches and can be seen as 'complex' [22].

Therefore, this research group designed a study under the hypothesis that a multidisciplinary intervention targeting identified characteristics of frailty would be effective in reducing frailty and improving functioning in frail older people [23].

Table 1. Principles of the FIT program

– Frailty can be mitigated
– Support needs to be individually tailored
– Intervention aims to improve physical, cognitive and social functioning
– Support has to be delivered over a long time period, and systems must facilitate consistent management
– Most frail older people should be encouraged and supported to adhere to their intervention plan
– It is important to recognize the needs of families and/or carers and to engage with them

Principles for Rehabilitation in Frailty

The FIT program was developed based on six underlying principles, which are summarized in table 1. First, frailty is seen as being treatable, or at least able to be mitigated. Second, the program to be provided needs to be individually tailored because frailty is a condition with components that vary according to the individual, and physical, cognitive and social functioning must be considered to address the broad range of issues that are involved. Support has to be provided over a long period of time to achieve the desired effects. Older people require assistance with adherence, which is likely to be difficult for them. Finally, the needs of family carers should be recognized. They should be engaged in the program, and their needs should also be met as part of the program.

The FIT program was conceptualized with the goal of tertiary prevention. People who are frail are assisted to address this transitional state and avoid complications of frailty. In particular, these complications are increased disability and the need for care, which may cause older people to leave their homes and move to an institutional setting.

Components of the Frailty Intervention Trial Program

The FIT program first identified the components of frailty that are present in individuals. The following five components of frailty are included in the Cardiovascular Health Study definition: unintentional weight loss, self-reported exhaustion, weakness, slow walking speed, and a low level of physical activity. It is difficult to measure some of these components in a clinical setting, particularly the physical activity level; thus, the strategy for assessing this criterion was modified in the FIT program [23].

Previous research and clinical studies have provided a strong evidence base for the technology of geriatric evaluation and management [12]. This technology was applied for each person participating in the FIT program, and in addition, the components of frailty applicable to each participant were targeted.

The lack of a cognitive dimension of the Cardiovascular Health Study definition of frailty was seen as a limitation. As a result, cognition was carefully assessed in each

Level of the ICF	Pattern of frailty	Common causes	Other causes
Health condition	Unstable health conditions	Infections, injuries, cardio respiratory disease	Frequent transition between primary care and acute hospital care
	Undernutrition*	Inability to prepare meals	Inability to purchase food Exhaustion
Impairment of structure/function	Psychological factors*	Depression, grief	Negative outlook
	Impaired cognition	Dementia	Lack of compensatory strategies
	Impaired vision/hearing	Macular degeneration, cataracts/presbycusis	Lack of appropriate equipment/ aids/eye surgery
Activity limitation	Decreased mobility*/ decreased self-care	Impaired balance and/or strength Environmental barriers	Decreased cardiovascular endurance Fear of falling
Participation restriction	Lack of participation in life roles	Social barriers Limited family contact Environmental barriers	Decreased self-efficacy
Environmental contextual factors	Problems with services or support systems	Services not readily available Lack of service co-ordination	Carer stress Interaction with support network Low income Physical or social isolation

* Captured in the frailty phenotype.

Adapted from Fairhall et al. [24].

Fig. 1. Important factors for assessing frail patients and the interactions between these factors.

frail person, and the intervention was tailored if cognitive impairment or dementia was present. People with severe cognitive impairment were excluded from the FIT program because the research group was unsure whether efficacy could be established in this context.

The paper 'Treating Frailty: a practical guide' [24] includes a detailed explanation of the FIT treatment approach. The FIT research group used the ICF to classify the common patterns present as part of, or in association with, frailty syndrome and identified their causes, which are outlined in figure 1. In summary, the common patterns were found to be related to health conditions, undernutrition, impaired cognition, vision or hearing problems, psychological factors, decreased mobility and self-care, a lack of participation in life roles, and problems with services or support systems. The FIT group identified and documented interventions and guidelines to address the common patterns of frailty in the clinical setting.

This group developed an assessment form, aiming to capture the data required to identify the common patterns of frailty and to plan interventions and a similar assessment form to guide the implementation of carer interventions [25].

The Frailty Intervention Trial Program: The Intervention

Details of the approach to planning interventions and to their implementations have been described elsewhere [23]. In summary, the frailty components as defined by Fried and colleagues, which were present in each participant, were specifically targeted. For all participants, additional interventions were provided or recommended based on CGA, including the management of chronic diseases, the treatment of pain, and the treatment of other identified syndromes or conditions, such as urinary incontinence.

The Frailty Intervention Trial Program: Information Processing

In the study evaluating the FIT program, there was a median of 10 face-to-face sessions with each participant, including a median of 8 sessions providing a strength, balance and endurance training program (the Weight-bearing Exercise for Better Balance (WEBB) program) [26]. In addition, there was a median of 4 telephone calls to each participant and a median of 4 telephone calls to other relevant parties.

The WEBB exercise program was delivered to 93% of the participants. A dietetic assessment and intervention were provided to 50% of the participants (and for 29% of the participants, nutritional supplements were recommended). A medical specialist consultation (geriatrics or rehabilitation medicine) was arranged for 24% of the participants, and only 3% were referred to a psychologist or psychiatrist.

A very broad range of additional interventions was provided as part of the frailty intervention, including the following (in the order of frequency, where frequency includes 20% or more of the participants): a liaison with the family, general practitioner (GP) and/or a service provider, 77%; an intervention targeting self-selected goals for participation in life roles, 51%; advice about footwear, 40%; modification of equipment, 34%; provision of equipment, 34%; a medication-related intervention, 33%; referral to the Aged Care Assessment Team [23], 31%; a telephone discussion with the GP about an urgent problem, 30%; referral to community transport, 25%; referral to a community nursing service, 23%; information on meal services, 24%; referral to an allied health service, 20%; and referral for follow-up of health conditions, 20%.

A standardized approach was used for the interventions in the study based on the study protocol and regular case discussions for each individual participant. In cases in which referrals were made to other health professionals and service providers, the treating physiotherapists provided reminders, when necessary, to ensure that the services were provided. More details of the interventions are provided in tables 2 and 3.

The Frailty Intervention Trial Program: Adherence

Adherence to the study protocol was documented by the physiotherapist who was primarily responsible for each participant. The global level of adherence (in the five categories) over the 12 months of the trial was estimated by the treating physiotherapist based on the following of the recommended interventions.

Adherence was 0% for 16 participants (13%), including 2 who died before the intervention commenced. Adherence levels of 1–25% were recorded for 34 (29%)

Table 2. Details of interventions directly targeting the Fried criteria (not all participants met each frailty criterion)

Fried criterion	Intervention (per FIT protocol)	Subjects receiving intervention	
		n	%
Slow walking	WEBB*	111	93
Weakness			
Weight loss	Dietician intervention	60	50
	Advice	60	50
	Nutritional supplements	35	29
	Others	7	6
Self-reported exhaustion	Referral to psychiatrist/psychologist	4	3
	Options to increase social engagement		
Self-reported exhaustion and reduced energy expenditure	Cognitive behavioral intervention		
	Working toward activity goals		
	Working toward participation goals	61	51
	Referral to services as necessary	120	100

* Weight-bearing Exercise for Better Balance exercise program [26].

participants, with 19 (16%) having 26–50% adherence, 52 (21%) attaining 51–75% adherence, and 25 (21%) achieving 76–100% adherence. Thus, the median overall adherence ranged from 26 to 50%.

Usual Care (Control) Group

The participants in the control group received the usual care available to older residents residing in the Hornsby Ku-ring-gai area from their GPs and provision of community services as determined by the GPs or other health or care providers.

The diaries of service use that were completed by all of the participants showed that both the usual care and intervention groups extensively used the health and care services. During the 12 months of follow-up, 9% of the participants died, 15% were admitted to nursing care facilities on a permanent basis, and 61% were hospitalized. Almost all of the participants utilized cleaning and housekeeping services.

Implementation of the Frailty Intervention Trial Program: Observations

Over the course of the study, the FIT group discerned different patterns of frailty and associated issues. From a clinical perspective, the following common patterns were observed: the 'physically' frail person, who is motivated and adherent to recommendations for treatment; the person who is frail and is also cognitively impaired; the frail

Table 3. Additional interventions that were delivered, some of which targeted the Fried criteria

	Intervention	Subjects	
		n	%
Liaison/triage	Liaison with GP, family, service provider	92	77
	Call GP for acute problem	36	30
	Arrange transport to hospital emergency department for acute problem	11	9
Equipment	Provide equipment	40	33
	Modify equipment	40	33
	Provide advice about footwear	48	40
	Recommend hip protectors (provided)	28 (4)	23 (3)
Medications	Intervention re: medications	39	33
	Calcium/vitamin D	4	3
	Community medication review	26	22
	Other medication advice	18	15
Carer support	Refer to Consultant for carer support	8	7
	Refer to Carers' Association/info pack	12	10
Link with services	Aged care assessment team	37	31
	Community transport	30	25
	Community nursing	28	23
	Info on meal services (excluding meals on wheels (MOW))	29	24
	Allied health (social work, physiotherapy, occupational therapy, hydrotherapy)	24	20
	MOW	14	12
	Day centers	13	11
	Taxi subsidy scheme	13	11
	Activities within residential care facility	12	10
	Hearing services	10	8
	Personal alarm	10	8
	Vision Australia or optometrist	8	7
	Podiatrist	8	7
	Orthotics/shoes	8	7
	Respite	7	6
	Disability parking scheme	5	4
	Continence clinic	6	5
	Memory clinic	3	3
	Gardening/mowing	3	3

person who is able to adhere to recommendations only to a limited extent; and the frail person with major psychological issues related to his or herself or the carer.

As an example, a woman who is 'physically' frail but is motivated and adherent to recommendations for treatment might participate in a rehabilitation program, including a progressive exercise program, input from a dietician with regard to a more nutritious diet, and household assistance for cleaning and shopping, in addition to contact with a geriatrician working with the program and a GP for rationalizing medications. At the conclusion of the program, no components of frailty syndrome, as defined by the Cardiovascular Health Study criteria, are present.

Results of the Frailty Intervention Trial Program

The FIT program was successful in achieving improvements in the primary outcomes, which included frailty (as defined by the Fried criteria) and physical functioning (as defined by the Short Physical Performance Battery) [27]. These results were reported together with analyses of the outcomes according to the level of adherence with the intervention [28].

In addition, there was a reduction in mobility-related disability in the program participants [29]. Further, there were some improvements in the statuses of the family carers [30].

In summary, the positive effects of the FIT program were evident after 12 months, and although trends toward improvement were present at 3 months, they were not statistically significant. These results support our contention and that of others [19] that programs aiming to improve functioning in older people have to be prolonged and moderately intensive. The number needed to treat for 12 months to reverse frailty in one person is 6.8. In comparison to other treatments, this number is very favorable.

The FIT group analyzed differences in components of the Fried frailty criteria after 12 months in the treatment group compared with the control group. There were statistically significant improvements in gait velocity and the level of physical activity, with a trend toward improvement in grip strength. No changes were detected in weight loss or exhaustion between the treatment groups.

There were no differences in the secondary outcomes as a result of the FIT program. A forthcoming publication will present incremental cost effectiveness ratios for this intervention, showing that for severely frail older people (those with four or five of the five Cardiovascular Health Study criteria), the FIT intervention is 'dominant', meaning that it is both less costly and more effective than usual care [31].

Interpreting the Results of the Frailty Intervention Trial Program

The FIT program's benefits became apparent at 12 months but were not evident at the 3-month follow-up. This finding shows that interventions treating frailty will most likely need to be prolonged. Supplementary analyses showed that the participants with higher levels of adherence to the interventions had much greater benefits after adjusting for possible confounders.

It was noted that initial improvements in frailty occurred in both the intervention and control groups, whereby 25% of the control participants became nonfrail by the

3-month follow-up. A likely explanation for this finding is that these individuals were still recovering from illness or injury when they entered the study. In the months before participating in the study, 73% of the participants had been hospitalized. It is noteworthy, however, that after 3 months, the frailty and mobility statuses of the intervention group were relatively stable, while those of the control group deteriorated.

Trials involving older people with reduced functioning who could be labeled as 'frail' have shown variable improvements in disability and its components. A systematic review of exercise interventions in frail populations has concluded that multicomponent exercise treatments for frail people are likely to be effective if they are undertaken on a regular basis over a prolonged period of time [19]. The geriatric evaluation and management literature has shown mixed effects with respect to the overall benefit of exercise [12].

In the FIT trial, it was not possible to blind the participants and treating clinicians to the intervention. The outcome assessors were blinded, but many of the participants inadvertently disclosed their treatment statuses. The components of the frailty definition were partly self-reported and partly performance-based, while one of the primary outcomes (the Short Physical Performance Battery) was a performance-based measure that should have reduced observer bias even when the assessor was unblinded.

The lack of a control group providing nonspecific contacts with the participants was seen as a limitation, and the trial did not reveal whether the nature of the contact is important. It is unlikely that such contacts have specific effects on frailty and mobility, but they could have affected mood, which may have influenced the exhaustion criterion of the Cardiovascular Health Study frailty phenotype [31]. However, the trial was pragmatic and was conducted as comparative effectiveness research for comparing the two options of usual care versus potential care through this program.

Adverse events were minor and responded to a change in the prescribed exercise intervention. Skilled physiotherapists were utilized to tailor and deliver the interventions. Drop-outs were not due to adverse events but were rather related to the participants' beliefs or to major changes in their health conditions.

There are limitations to the generalizability of this approach because the study was conducted in a relatively affluent country with well-developed health and care services for older people. Further, a specific clinical team with considerable experience and knowledge of the locally available aged care services was utilized. However, it should be feasible to generalize the intervention to other situations and contexts with similar health and care services. This moderate intensity intervention could be provided as a program through an aged care health service. It costs about a quarter of the amount of the program currently administered by the Australian government, which was designed to assist a similar group of older people with the transition from the hospital to the home or nursing care facility [32].

In the group studied, it was difficult to distinguish 'frailty' from 'disability' because these two states coexisted in almost all of the participants. While improvements in frailty were seen, there were also improvements in mobility disability. The changes in frailty and mobility were similar in magnitude and represented medium effect sizes. In this study, the changes in frailty and mobility appeared to be closely linked.

This study has shown that treating frailty in older people is a realistic therapeutic goal. Ideally, a multi-center study with a larger sample size should be conducted to confirm and extend the findings of this study. Future studies should also consider follow-ups beyond the end of the intervention period. The findings of the FIT program of frailty rehabilitation need to be replicated in similar populations of frail older people who live in other settings, particularly communities with different health and care systems. The costs of this tertiary frailty prevention program also need to be assessed in more detail.

Conclusion

Rehabilitation approaches to frailty are in the early stages of development. However, there are clear theoretical reasons to expect that a rehabilitation approach will be effective. In addition, some experimental data are available suggesting that rehabilitation is effective in frail and pre-frail older people.

Frailty shows promise as a prognostic indicator for rehabilitation programs in a similar manner to its application in other areas of medicine. However, care should be taken not to exclude frail older people from rehabilitation, as has been the case at some centers for people with cognitive impairment or very severe disability.

References

1 Australasian Rehabilitation Outcomes Centre: AROC Ambulatory National Report. January 2012 – December 2012. Australasian Faculty of Rehabilitation Medicine and University of Wollongong, 2012.
2 Halbert J, Crotty M, Whitehead C, Cameron I, Kurrle S, Graham S, et al: Multi-disciplinary rehabilitation after hip fracture is associated with improved outcome: a systematic review. J Rehabil Med 2007; 39:507–512.
3 Pollock A, Baer G, Campbell P, Choo PL, Forster A, Morris J, et al: Physical rehabilitation approaches for the recovery of function and mobility following stroke. Cochrane Database Syst Rev 2014;4: CD001920.
4 Singh I, Gallacher J, Davis K, Johansen A, Eeles E, Hubbard RE: Predictors of adverse outcomes on an acute geriatric rehabilitation ward. Age Ageing 2012; 41:242–246.
5 World Health Organization (WHO): The International Classification of Functioning, Disability and Health. Geneva, WHO, 2001.
6 Landefeld CS, Palmer RM, Kresevic DM, Fortinsky RH, Kowal J: A randomized trial of care in a hospital medical unit especially designed to improve the functional outcomes of acutely ill older patients. N Engl J Med 1995;332:1338–1344.
7 Morley JE, Vellas B, van Kan GA, Anker SD, Bauer JM, Bernabei R, et al: Frailty consensus: a call to action. J Am Med Dir Assoc 2013;14:392–397.
8 World Health Organization (WHO): World Report on Disability. Geneva, WHO, 2011.
9 Buchner DM, Larson EB, Wagner EH, Koepsell TD, de Lateur BJ: Evidence for a non-linear relationship between leg strength and gait speed. Age Ageing 1996;25:386–391.
10 World Health Organization (WHO): The International Classification of Health Interventions. http://www.who.int/classifications/ichi/en/ (accessed May 24, 2014).
11 Stuck AE, Iliffe S: Comprehensive geriatric assessment for older adults. BMJ 2011;343:d6799.

12 Stuck AE, Siu AL, Wieland GD, Adams J, Rubenstein LZ: Comprehensive geriatric assessment: a meta-analysis of controlled trials. Lancet 1993;342:1032–1036.
13 Robinson TN, Wu DS, Pointer L, Dunn CL, Cleveland JC Jr, Moss M: Simple frailty score predicts postoperative complications across surgical specialties. Am J Surg 2013;206:544–550.
14 Aaldriks AA, Giltay EJ, le Cessie S, van der Geest LG, Portielje JE, Tanis BC, et al: Prognostic value of geriatric assessment in older patients with advanced breast cancer receiving chemotherapy. Breast 2013;22:753–760.
15 Kawryshanker S, Raymond W, Ingram K, Inderjeeth CA: Effect of frailty on functional gain, resource utilisation, and discharge destination: an observational prospective study in a GEM ward. Curr Gerontol Geriatr Res 2014;2014:357857.
16 Krishnan M, Beck S, Havelock W, Eeles E, Hubbard RE, Johansen A: Predicting outcome after hip fracture: using a frailty index to integrate comprehensive geriatric assessment results. Age Ageing 2014;43:122–126.
17 Collaborative systematic review of the randomised trials of organised inpatient (stroke unit) care after stroke. Stroke Unit Trialists' Collaboration. BMJ 1997;314:1151–1159.
18 Beswick AD, Rees K, Dieppe P, Ayis S, Gooberman-Hill R, Horwood J, et al: Complex interventions to improve physical function and maintain independent living in elderly people: a systematic review and meta-analysis. Lancet 2008;371:725–735.
19 Theou O, Stathokostas L, Roland KP, Jakobi JM, Patterson C, Vandervoort AA, et al: The effectiveness of exercise interventions for the management of frailty: a systematic review. J Aging Res 2011;2011:569194.
20 Drey M, Zech A, Freiberger E, Bertsch T, Uter W, Sieber CC, et al: Effects of strength training versus power training on physical performance in prefrail community-dwelling older adults. Gerontology 2012;58:197–204.
21 Pre-FIT: the effects of an interdisciplinary multifactorial intervention versus usual care on pre-frailty and mobility function in pre frail older people. Trial ID: ACTRN12613000043730. Australian New Zealand Clinical Trials Registry, 2013. https://www.anzctr.org.au/Trial/Registration/TrialReview.aspx?id=363480 (accessed May 24, 2014).
22 Craig P, Dieppe P, Macintyre S, Michie S, Nazareth I, Petticrew M, et al: Developing and evaluating complex interventions: the new Medical Research Council guidance. BMJ 2008;337:a1655.
23 Fairhall N, Aggar C, Kurrle SE, Sherrington C, Lord S, Lockwood K, et al: Frailty Intervention Trial (FIT). BMC Geriatr 2008;8:27.
24 Fairhall N, Langron C, Sherrington C, Lord SR, Kurrle SE, Lockwood K, et al: Treating frailty-a practical guide. BMC Med 2011;9:83.
25 Cameron ID, Aggar C, Robinson AL, Kurrle SE: Assessing and helping carers of older people. BMJ 2011;343:d5202.
26 Weight-bearing Exercise for Better Balance (WEBB). http://www.webb.org.au/ (accessed May 24, 2014).
27 Guralnik JM, Simonsick EM, Ferrucci L, Glynn RJ, Berkman LF, Blazer DG, et al: A short physical performance battery assessing lower extremity function: association with self-reported disability and prediction of mortality and nursing home admission. J Gerontol 1994;49:M85–M94.
28 Cameron ID, Fairhall N, Langron C, Lockwood K, Monaghan N, Aggar C, et al: A multifactorial interdisciplinary intervention reduces frailty in older people: randomized trial. BMC Med 2013;11:65.
29 Fairhall N, Sherrington C, Kurrle SE, Lord SR, Lockwood K, Cameron ID: Effect of a multifactorial interdisciplinary intervention on mobility-related disability in frail older people: randomised controlled trial. BMC Med 2012;10:120.
30 Aggar C, Ronaldson S, Cameron ID: Reactions to caregiving during an intervention targeting frailty in community living older people. BMC Geriatr 2012;12:66.
31 Fairhall N, Sherrington C, Kurrle SE, Lord SR, Lockwood K, Howard K, et al: Economic evaluation of a multi-factorial, interdisciplinary intervention versus usual care to reduce frailty in frail older people. J Am Med Dir Assoc 2015;16:41–48.
32 Hall CJ, Peel NM, Comans TA, Gray LC, Scuffham PA: Can post-acute care programmes for older people reduce overall costs in the health system? A case study using the Australian Transition Care Programme. Health Soc Care Community 2012;20:97–102.

Prof. Ian D. Cameron
John Walsh Centre for Rehabilitation Research, Sydney Medical School Northern
Kolling Institute of Medical Research, Royal North Shore Hospital
St Leonards, NSW 2065 (Australia)
E-Mail ian.cameron@sydney.edu.au

Theou O, Rockwood K (eds): Frailty in Aging. Biological, Clinical and Social Implications.
Interdiscipl Top Gerontol Geriatr. Basel, Karger, 2015, vol 41, pp 151–160 (DOI: 10.1159/000381232)

End of Life Care in Frailty

Paige Moorhouse · Katalin Koller · Laurie Mallery
Dalhousie University, Halifax, N.S., Canada

Abstract
The increasing prevalence of frailty within the aging population poses challenges to current models of chronic disease management and end-of-life care delivery. As frailty progresses, individuals face an increasing frequency of acute health issues requiring medical attention. The ability of health care systems to recognize and respond to acute health issues in frail patients using a holistic understanding of health and prognosis will play a central role in ensuring their effective and appropriate care, including that at the end of their lives. This chapter reviews the history of palliative care and the elements of frailty that require the modification of current models of palliative care. In addition, tools and models for recognition of end of life in frailty and considerations for symptom management are introduced.

To deliver effective end-of-life care when frailty is present, the paradigms of traditional palliative care need modification to address important differences between younger and older individuals. In contrast to younger cancer patients, who typically have predominant single-system diseases, the majority of frail older adults die with complex interacting chronic medical illnesses and symptoms [1]. To appreciate the unique challenges that frailty poses to optimal end-of-life care, it is first useful to understand the history and evolution of modern palliative care paradigms. Palliative care began in the 1960s with the hospice movement, which was spearheaded in the United Kingdom by Dame Cicely Saunders and her American protégé, Florence Wald. Following her studies of philosophy at Oxford, Dame Saunders became a Red Cross nurse during World War II. When she worked at St. Thomas' Hospital, she observed that many health care providers were uncomfortable with death and were reluctant to provide relief for what she termed 'total pain' – the culmination of physical, emotional, social and spiritual distress. In her letters, Dame Saunders described her concern for patients who were not informed of their prognosis and for those who experienced profound suffering at the end of life.

'It seems inevitable that a backlash to such blind optimism would arise… the power of belief in the cult of cure was so strong that it denied the very existence of dying patients as a class of people. Deaths, if they occurred, were aberrations; in the cult of cure people did not die, they coded' [2].

Her acknowledgment of death as a life stage through which we all travel was later captured by her choice of St. Christopher's (the patron saint of travelers) as the name of the first hospice mission in 1967 after she became a physician. Today, hospice care includes inpatient and home care services for those who are nearing the end of life and are often in the last 6 months of life. Following Dame Saunders' revolutionary work and the establishment of hospice care, palliative care was developed as a medical subspecialty. Palliative care is an umbrella term that refers to medical care for serious illnesses, focusing on symptom relief, emotional and psychosocial support, optimization of quality of life, and end-of-life planning. It can be provided to any patient regardless of the prognosis or disease state. In contrast to end-of-life care, palliative care can be delivered concurrently with treatment directed at a cure. As the population ages, progressive chronic conditions, such as obstructive lung disease and dementia, will equally require timely palliative interventions [3]. However, when multiple health issues culminate in frailty, standard models of palliative care can present challenges to optimal care at the end of life. Therefore, at this moment in time, we face similar challenges to those that were identified by Dame Saunders in the 1960s.

Challenges to Optimal End-of-Life Care Delivery in Frailty

The first challenge to the delivery of optimal end-of-life care in frailty is the single-system illness model, which is the basis for the delivery of much of specialized medicine, including palliative care [4]. When frailty is present, the model of addressing 'one thing at once' often leads to an inadequate understanding of the interaction between chronic illnesses and their effects on quality of life. For example, effective guidelines and models for end-of-life care for chronic obstructive lung disease have been developed, but the applicability of such guidelines is challenged when there are multiple, competing causes of symptoms and mortality [5]. Further, clinical practice guidelines designed for specific diseases are often based on studies that did not enroll frail older adults. As such, some of the recommended treatments may be ineffective, too difficult to manage, or intolerable due to adverse effects. Similarly, the single system disease model often compounds the complexity of frailty because each issue is addressed with a specialty-based focus, which results in multiple specialized assessments and recommendations with little attention to the high-level integration of the results of such assessments [4]. The Achilles heel of the single-system illness model is the related challenge of recognizing end of life in frail patients. Although frailty has been robustly associated with poor health outcomes across populations and clinical settings, it has yet to be measured as part of routine care in most clinical settings. The working definitions and measurement tools for frailty are reviewed elsewhere in this book, and there is disagreement as to the optimal measure to use for care planning. Regardless of how frailty is defined or measured, it is associated with vulnerability to poor health outcomes that matter to patients, including mortality, morbidity, length of hospital stay, functional decline, adverse drug reactions and falls [6–11].

In the absence of the routine identification and measurement of frailty, many frail patients with advanced and incurable diseases receive highly aggressive interventions that have little chance of success and result in prolonged suffering before death [4, 12]. By its very nature, frailty is associated with heterogeneity and uncertainty in terms of future health. Significantly, clinicians identify uncertainty in prognosis as an impediment to effective communication with patients [13]. However, universal truths related to frailty, including its evident progression and its association with the end of life in cases of severe frailty, underscore the important role of careful care planning.

Clinicians have several tools at their disposal to aid in the recognition of approaching end of life in frailty, ranging from quick screening tools to more in-depth assessments. In addition to screening tools for frailty, a useful rapid screen is the following 'surprise' question for clinician self-reflection: 'Would you be surprised if this patient died within the next year?' [14]. This question is a powerful antidote to the reluctance of clinicians to estimate life expectancy by instead asking them to acknowledge that there is a risk of death. An answer to this 'surprise' question indicating that death would not be unexpected or a 'surprise' highlights an opportunity for the clinician to carefully review the care plan and to acknowledge the diminishing role of interventions designed to reduce long-term risk, such as preventative health measures.

A more detailed assessment of the drivers of frailty can be completed using comprehensive geriatric assessment [15], which is a well-studied and validated methodology whereby clinicians assess the overall health of patients by determining details (and trajectory of change) in the domains of cognition, mood, motivation, mobility, activities of daily living, social circumstances, co-morbidities and medications. When using comprehensive geriatric assessment in populations in which cognitive impairment and functional dependence are common, gathering history from a collateral source helps clinicians to develop a more complete understanding of the health picture. Beyond improving a clinician's understanding of a patient's overall health, the experience of history-taking from a collateral source in relation to the patient's day-to-day functioning and cognition can be an important part of building rapport with the patient's caregiver and validating their experience. Here again, Dame Saunders quietly developed a strategy in which the understanding of the patient's story becomes part of the treatment:

> 'All [work] should stem from respect for the patient and very close attention to his distress. It means really looking at him, learning what this kind of pain is like, what these symptoms are like, and from this knowledge finding out how best to relieve them. We have to learn what it feels like to be so ill, to be leaving life and its activity, to know that your faculties are failing, that you are parting from loves and responsibilities. We have to learn how to feel "with" patients without feeling "like" them if we are to give the kind of listening and steady support that they need to find their own way through' [16].

While Dame Saunders originally intended to apply this decree to *patients*, those who are frail become increasingly reliant upon others, and involvement of the caregivers of patients ensures a feasible and informed approach to care planning. Armed with a 360-degree snapshot of a patient's baseline cognition, function and mobility and how he or she has changed over time, a clinician can recognize markers of severe frailty that may include the following [17]:

- dependence on others for hands-on assistance with basic activities of daily living;
- severe-stage dementia;
- profound social isolation or the lack of an available or reliable caregiver; and
- a new inability to ambulate without the assistance of another person.

When severe frailty is present, several features of the patient history can be helpful in identifying poor prognosis [4]. These include the following: a gradual and unrelenting decline in physical and cognitive functioning, unexplained weight loss and an increasing frequency of acute health crises associated with incomplete functional recovery. These features present an opportunity for the clinician to consider that the end of life may be approaching. The third challenge to the delivery of optimal end-of-life care in frailty is the high prevalence of cognitive impairment among severely frail older adults. Although cognitive impairment is an important driver of frailty, dementia remains an under-diagnosed entity in community and institutional settings [18, 19]. Notably, advanced dementia has a mortality risk comparable to most cancers and is associated with considerable morbidity, including increased risks of delirium during hospitalization and functional decline following hospitalization [20, 21].

Although caregivers may be aware of memory issues, they are often uninformed about the degree, scope, and implications of cognitive impairment as they relate to future health and treatment choices [22]. Therefore, diagnosing dementia presents an important opportunity to optimally engage patients and/or their caregivers in the care planning process, to anticipate common health crises that occur in advanced dementia, such as pneumonia and hip fracture, and to contextualize all health care planning decisions within the framework of a progressive, incurable disease.

The presence and degree of frailty have important implications for decision making in dementia. For example, for patient with dementia and frailty, the presence of chronic health issues associated with acute exacerbations and shortened life expectancy, such as chronic obstructive lung disease or congestive heart failure, provide an opportunity to develop a crisis care plan that balances baseline quality of life (the quality of life enjoyed prior to the exacerbation) with the inherent risks of incomplete cognitive and functional recovery associated with hospitalization or aggressive medical interventions. When dementia is present, care planning must always consider the possible impact of treatment on cognition, including the risks of worsening cognition due to the incomplete recovery of delirium, intensification of behavioral issues, and institutionalization. Further, the successful treatment of curable health issues will increase the likelihood of survival to progress through the stages of dementia – an outcome that may not be acceptable to all patients.

The fourth challenge to optimal end-of-life care in frailty is the paralyzing effect of uncertainty. The heterogeneity of the patient experience and that of the phenotype of frailty are associated with considerable prognostic uncertainty. Clinicians admit that uncertainty in prognosis often leads to aversion to discussing the implications of frailty [13, 23]. However, a better understanding of frailty is a critical first step because patients and families have indicated that the degree to which their expectations are aligned with the natural history of a disease plays a key role in their satisfaction and comfort with end-of-life care [24]. Further, although clinicians may be reluctant to develop and present their clinical opinions, most patients and families appreciate guidance and recommendations that are based on evidence as well as clinical judgment [25]. Clinicians must develop comfort with the complexity and uncertainty that comes with frailty at the end of life and acknowledge that some outcomes may be unpredictable. Nevertheless, because of the phenomenology and natural history of frailty, some certainties can be communicated. For example, frail older adults are more at risk for transition to end of life compared to older adults who are healthy. Similarly, although the timing and nature will vary, all frail older adults can expect to experience a 'health crisis' – an acute worsening of health due to the exacerbation of an existing health issue or the development of a new health issue that requires medical attention [26]. Finally, health crises in frailty commonly result in functional or cognitive decline with incomplete recovery, a possibility that increases with more advanced frailty [4]. Notably, a history of prior incomplete functional and/or cognitive recovery can be used to help patients and caregivers understand the implications of future health crises. These three certainties of frailty – the shortened life expectancy, the inevitable decline in health, and the potential for worsening health following acute illness – indicate that as severely frail older adults transition to the end of life, they can expect to experience a gradual decline in overall health, typically punctuated by episodes of acute decline and incomplete recovery. With this in mind, baseline quality of life prior to the health crisis can clarify the risk/benefit tradeoffs of medical and surgical interventions.

Symptom Management in Frailty

As frailty progresses, the indication for a palliative focus increases. Symptom relief and optimizing quality of life remain the backbone of palliation because symptom burden is often high in the presence of significant frailty. Comorbidities can compound symptom severity and often require an approach that balances medication benefits with adverse effects in a population in which treatments may be ineffective or poorly tolerated. For example, effective pain relief may be limited by the sedative or cognitive side effects of a medication, and the behavioral problems of dementia may be unresponsive to pharmacological and nonpharmacological therapies [27]. Further, symptom assessment can be difficult due to communication barriers related to dementia. These challenges must be addressed to avoid the under- and over-treatment of symptoms, particularly pain.

With palliative care in the presence of frailty, the geriatric paradigm 'start low and go slow' should be followed by 'but go!' to underscore the need to effectively reach therapeutic targets, when possible, so that under-treatment is avoided. Periodic medication reviews can ensure that medications are being used to optimize quality of life, rather than to endorse medications that are unlikely to provide benefit at the end of life. In addition to updating symptom burden, medication reviews should make recommendations to discontinue ineffective or unnecessary medications, minimize potential drug interactions, and manage the total medication burden [28]. It may also be prudent to stop medications that are causing symptoms. For example, discontinuing an angiotensin-converting enzyme inhibitor in a patient with elevated seated systolic blood pressure, but with orthostasis and falls, can be viewed as a focus on symptom control rather than on trying to achieve cardioprotection, particularly in the setting of limited life expectancy. Other symptoms commonly encountered in dementia, such as dysphagia and behavioral problems, also need to be carefully managed using strategies that consider the effect of each treatment on quality of life. This recommendation is particularly important in the presence of symptoms such as gastroparesis or dysphagia, which are commonly encountered in patients with advanced dementia [29].

Pain may be under-assessed and under-treated in older patients, particularly in the setting of dementia [29]. Clinicians should strive to take a full symptom inventory, even when verbal communication is hindered. Nonverbal pain scales and collateral symptom history from a reliable informant can help with this process and with symptom monitoring once treatment has commenced [30]. Pain should always be considered when confronting the emergence or intensification of behavioral symptoms [31].

Opioids remain a cornerstone treatment for pain and dyspnea. When using opioids, vigilant monitoring of cognitive effects and bowel function is essential. A routine bowel regimen should commence concurrently and be adjusted accordingly. Optimization of nonopioid analgesics can assist in reducing the total daily opioid dose required to reach the therapeutic target. Acetaminophen, used regularly throughout the day within dosing guidelines, is generally regarded as a first-line pain medication in older adults before nonsteroidal anti-inflammatory drugs, which have potential renal, cardiac and gastrointestinal side effects.

Adjunctive analgesic modalities can play supportive roles in symptom control for frail patients, helping to limit higher doses of medication. When an nonsteroidal anti-inflammatory drug is being considered, the regulated use of a topical preparation may reduce systemic effects [29], although efficacy is modest, and systemic side effects are still possible. With judicious monitoring to ensure tolerance, anticonvulsants and antidepressants, particularly tricyclic antidepressants, may be trialed to treat neuropathic pain [29]. Nonpharmacologic strategies, such as massage therapy, acupuncture, hydrotherapy and hot and cold packs, may also provide pain relief [32].

The clinical and pharmacokinetic correlates of frailty also merit consideration when palliation of gastrointestinal symptoms is required. As with other symptoms, medication reviews can identify medications that are at least partly responsible. For example, drugs that can cause constipation, such as iron supplements and calcium, may be culprits. In the nonfrail population, nausea can be treated with antinauseant medications that target specific emetic pathways. In frail patients, potential adverse effects herald a need for extra caution. For example, steroids may be used to treat nausea but may be associated with intolerable insomnia, anxiety or delirium in frail patients. Dopamine antagonists, such as haloperidol and other neuroleptic medications, may unmask or exacerbate parkinsonism, although the potential extrapyramidal symptoms vary based on each drug's receptor activity. Anticholinergic medications, such as dimenhydrinate, can worsen cognition. Nonpharmacologic environmental modifications may be useful in the management of nausea. Examples include avoiding strong odors, offering small, attractive meals and providing cool, carbonated beverages.

It is also important to address emotional symptoms when providing comprehensive palliative care. Anxiety and impaired mood can directly impact pain control [33]. Consultation with allied health care providers, including social workers and spiritual care providers, can help patients and families to manage physiosocial stressors using a comprehensive palliative care plan.

What Is Needed to Move Health Care Providers and Systems Forward in the Provision of End-of-Life Care in Frailty?

Similar to the experience of Dame Saunders in the 1960s, our current health care system is at a crossroads at which the ability to question and remediate routines of care that hamper the spiritual and comfortable deaths of frail older adults will determine whether and to what degree our system is able to respond and evolve.

The Palliative and Therapeutic Harmonization (PATH) program is one example of a transdisciplinary approach to frailty that advances the recognition of and response to terminal frailty through standardized assessment and treatment protocols that align goals of care with prognosis. This program includes a three-step process with the following aims:

(1) to enhance the capacities of health care teams and individuals for producing an organized and coherent picture of health status based on the understanding of each person's cognition, mobility, function, social situation, and health conditions;

(2) to foster information exchange between patients/families and health care workers to improve the collective appreciation of health status and prognosis based on underlying health conditions; and

(3) to empower patients/families and health care workers to consider present and future health status, as well as the holistic vulnerability associated with frailty, when making medical and personal care decisions.

These three steps aim to remedy many of the obstacles described above that commonly take place when attempting to provide good palliative care to older adults who are frail. The first step, identifying frailty, makes use of a frailty screen or standardized assessment to define functional, cognitive, and health statuses. Identifying a collateral historian and documenting their perception of functional and cognitive abilities is an essential part of this process. Understanding frailty burden allows health professionals to anticipate the impact of each condition and its proposed treatment on overall health.

The second step in the PATH model calls for methodical communication as a distinct and essential process to help patients and/or families understand that frailty shortens life, worsens over time and is associated with vulnerability to negative health outcomes. Communication is completed using semi-structured interviews that review each health issue and its expected worsening. For example, if Alzheimer-type dementia is present, the current stage and typical progression of the illness is described, usually to the substitute decision-maker. This communication process improves the understanding of the patient's health and allows individuals to make health care decisions that appropriately consider the background of frailty. This step is compatible with available evidence that shows that giving detailed information to patients or their substitute decision-makers can significantly change the types of decisions that are made [34].

The guided information exchange in the second step of PATH aims to help individuals understand that complex medical treatments that work well for healthier individuals may have a different risk-benefit trade-off in those who are frail because there may be fewer years of life to experience treatment benefits should they occur and greater risks. Decision-making discussions focus less on calculating life expectancy and more significantly on how to make immediate treatment decisions (such as whether to pursue surgery for symptomatic aortic stenosis) and how to deal with health crises that will inevitably occur, such as future episodes of pneumonia, hip fracture, or worsening health. The intended outcome is not to impose rigid directives into the dynamic process of frailty, but rather to allow those patients who are severely or very severely frail to avoid treatments or interventions that are inconsistent with the goals of care. This process also readies health professionals to deal with future crises through better care planning.

The use of the PATH process improves appropriateness of care, with one study demonstrating that its application resulted in a 75% reduction in the demand for interventional treatments for significantly frail patients [26]. Controlling for age, those with higher baseline frailty were more likely to decline scheduled interventions (odds ratio (OR) = 3.41, 95% confidence interval (CI) = 1.39–8.38). Similarly, those with later-stage dementia (according to the Functional Assessment Staging Tool score) [61] more commonly declined previously scheduled interventions (OR = 1.66, 95% CI = 1.05–2.65) compared to those with earlier-stage or no dementia.

The PATH program has also developed several clinical practice guidelines that consider frailty for common chronic health conditions, such as diabetes, hypertension, and hyperlipidemia [35]. These guidelines provide guidance on how to liberalize treatment targets to balance risk and benefit and present new standards for treating older adults who are frail.

Conclusion

After forging more holistic and compassionate end-of-life care strategies for patients with cancer, Dame Cicely Saunders died of cancer in 2005 at the age of 87 at St. Christopher's Hospice. Even in her death, Dame Saunders provides a powerful example and message. The discipline of geriatric medicine has much to learn and much to teach with regard to recognizing end of life due to frailty. Only then can patients and their families be empowered to experience the very kind of death that we would hope to experience ourselves.

References

1 Burge F, Johnston G, Lawson B, Dewar R, Cummings I: Population-based trends in referral of the elderly to a comprehensive palliative care programme. Palliat Med 2002;16:255–256.
2 Hallenbeck J: Palliative care in the final days of life: 'they were expecting it at any time'. JAMA 2005;293: 2265–2271.
3 Koller K, Rockwood K: Frailty in older adults: implications for end-of-life care. Cleve Clin J Med 2013; 80:168–174.
4 Mallery LH, Moorhouse P: Respecting frailty. J Med Ethics 2011;37:126–128.
5 Rocker GM, Cook D: 'INSPIRED' approaches to better care for patients with advanced COPD. Clin Invest Med 2013;36:E114–E120.
6 Ekerstad N, Swahn E, Janzon M, Alfredsson J, Lofmark R, Lindenberger M, Carlsson P: Frailty is independently associated with short-term outcomes for elderly patients with non-ST-segment elevation myocardial infarction. Circulation 2011;124:2397–2404.
7 Fried LP, Kronmal RA, Newman AB, Bild DE, Mittelmark MB, Polak JF, Robbins JA, Gardin JM: Risk factors for 5-year mortality in older adults: the Cardiovascular Health Study. JAMA 1998;279:585–592.
8 Johansen KL, Chertow GM, Jin C, Kutner NG: Significance of frailty among dialysis patients. J Am Soc Nephrol 2007;18:2960–2967.
9 Lee DH, Buth KJ, Martin BJ, Yip AM, Hirsch GM: Frail patients are at increased risk for mortality and prolonged institutional care after cardiac surgery. Circulation 2010;121:973–978.
10 Makary MA, Segev DL, Pronovost PJ, Syin D, Bandeen-Roche K, Patel P, Takenaga R, Devgan L, Holzmueller CG, Tian J, Fried LP: Frailty as a predictor of surgical outcomes in older patients. J Am Coll Surg 2010;210:901–908.
11 Mitnitski AB, Mogilner AJ, MacKnight C, Rockwood K: The mortality rate as a function of accumulated deficits in a frailty index. Mech Ageing Dev 2002;123:1457–1460.
12 Smith AK, Cenzer IS, Knight SJ, Puntillo KA, Widera E, Williams BA, Boscardin WJ, Covinsky KE: The epidemiology of pain during the last 2 years of life. Ann Intern Med 2010;153:563–569.
13 Hancock K, Clayton JM, Parker SM, Wal der S, Butow PN, Carrick S, Currow D, Ghersi D, Glare P, Hagerty R, Tattersall MH: Truth-telling in discussing prognosis in advanced life-limiting illnesses: a systematic review. Palliat Med 2007;21:507–517.
14 Johnson DC, Kutner JS, Armstrong JD 2nd: Would you be surprised if this patient died? Preliminary exploration of first and second year residents' approach to care decisions in critically ill patients. BMC Palliat Care 2003;2:1.
15 Ellis G, Whitehead MA, Robinson D, O'Neill D, Langhorne P: Comprehensive geriatric assessment for older adults admitted to hospital: meta-analysis of randomised controlled trials. BMJ 2011;343: d6553.
16 Saunders C: 'Watch with me'. Nurs Times 1965;61: 1615–1617.

17 Rockwood K, Song X, MacKnight C, Bergman H, Hogan DB, McDowell I, Mitnitski A: A global clinical measure of fitness and frailty in elderly people. CMAJ 2005;173:489–495.
18 Barton C, Miller B, Yaffe K: Improved evaluation and management of cognitive impairment: results of a comprehensive intervention in long-term care. J Am Med Dir Assoc 2006;7:84–89.
19 Sternberg SA, Wolfson C, Baumgarten M: Undetected dementia in community-dwelling older people: the Canadian Study of Health and Aging. J Am Geriatr Soc 2000;48:1430–1434.
20 Cole MG, Ciamp A, Belzile E, Zhong L: Persistent delirium in older hospital patients: a systematic review of frequency and prognosis. Age Ageing 2009; 38:19–26.
21 Orsitto G, Cascavilla L, Franceschi M, Aloia RM, Greco A, Paris F, Seripa D, Pilotto A: Influence of cognitive impairment and comorbidity on disability in hospitalized elderly patients. J Nutr Health Aging 2005;9:194–198.
22 Moorhouse P: Care planning in dementia: tips for clinicians. Neurodegener Dis Manag 2014;4:57–66.
23 Sullivan AM, Lakoma MD, Matsuyama RK, Rosenblatt L, Arnold RM, Block SD: Diagnosing and discussing imminent death in the hospital: a secondary analysis of physician interviews. J Palliat Med 2007; 10:882–893.
24 van der Steen JT, Onwuteaka-Philipsen BD, Knol DL, Ribbe MW, Deliens L: Caregivers' understanding of dementia predicts patients' comfort at death: a prospective observational study. BMC Med 2013; 11:105.
25 Roland M, Paddison C: Better management of patients with multimorbidity. BMJ 2013;346:f2510.
26 Moorhouse P, Mallery LH: Palliative and therapeutic harmonization: a model for appropriate decision-making in frail older adults. J Am Geriatr Soc 2012; 60:2326–2332.
27 Schneider LS, Tariot PN, Dagerman KS, Davis SM, Hsiao JK, Ismail MS, Lebowitz BD, Lyketsos CG, Ryan JM, Stroup TS, Sultzer DL, Weintraub D, Lieberman JA: Effectiveness of atypical antipsychotic drugs in patients with Alzheimer's disease. N Engl J Med 2006;355:1525–1538.
28 Holmes HM, Hayley DC, Alexander GC, Sachs GA: Reconsidering medication appropriateness for patients late in life. Arch Intern Med 2006;166:605–609.
29 American Geriatrics Society Panel on Pharmacological Management of Persistent Pain in Older Persons: Pharmacological management of persistent pain in older persons. J Am Geriatr Soc 2009;57: 1331–1346.
30 Kapo J, Morrison LJ, Liao S: Palliative care for the older adult. J Palliat Med 2007;10:185–209.
31 Hersch EC, Falzgraf S: Management of the behavioral and psychological symptoms of dementia. Clin Interv Aging 2007;2:611–621.
32 Abdulla A, Adams N, Bone M, Elliott AM, Gaffin J, Jones D, Knaggs R, Martin D, Sampson L, Schofield P: Guidance on the management of pain in older people. Age Ageing 2013;42(suppl 1):i1–i57.
33 Ryan T, Ingleton C, Gardiner C, Parker C, Gott M, Noble B: Symptom burden, palliative care need and predictors of physical and psychological discomfort in two UK hospitals. BMC Palliat Care 2013;12:11.
34 Volandes AE, Paasche-Orlow MK, Barry MJ, Gillick MR, Minaker KL, Chang Y, Cook EF, Abbo ED, El-Jawahri A, Mitchell SL: Video decision support tool for advance care planning in dementia: randomised controlled trial. BMJ 2009;338:b2159.
35 Mallery LH, Ransom T, Steeves B, Cook B, Dunbar P, Moorhouse P: Evidence-informed guidelines for treating frail older adults with type 2 diabetes: from the Diabetes Care Program of Nova Scotia (DCPNS) and the Palliative and Therapeutic Harmonization (PATH) program. J Am Med Dir Assoc 2013;14: 801–808.

Paige Moorhouse, MD, MPH, FRCPC
Dalhousie University
Suite 1308, Veterans' Memorial Building, 5595 Veteran's Memorial Lane
Halifax, NS B2H2P1 (Canada)
E-Mail paige.moorhouse@cdha.nshealth.ca

Theou O, Rockwood K (eds): Frailty in Aging. Biological, Clinical and Social Implications.
Interdiscipl Top Gerontol Geriatr. Basel, Karger, 2015, vol 41, pp 161–173 (DOI: 10.1159/000381233)

Frailty and Organization of Health and Social Care

Andrew Clegg · John Young

Academic Unit of Elderly Care and Rehabilitation, University of Leeds, Leeds, UK

Abstract

In this chapter, we consider how health and social care can best be organized for older people with frailty. We will consider the merits of routine frailty identification, including risk stratification methods, to inform the provision of evidence-based treatment and holistic, goal-oriented care. We will also consider how best to place older people with frailty at the heart of health and social care systems so that the complex challenges associated with this vulnerable group are addressed.

Older people with frailty are majority users of many health and social care services [1]. Older people, and particularly those with frailty, account for the majority of hospital bed days and adult social care spending in higher-income countries [2]. However, modern health care systems are mostly organized around single-system illnesses more typically found in younger people, rather than in older people with frailty [3]. Frail older people are vulnerable to major changes in health following minor illness, resulting in the common presentations of mobility impairment, delirium and falls. These symptoms, although the consequence of an acute medical illness, may not be perceived as such, and pejorative terms such as 'acopia' have been used. Resources, clinical priorities and research funding are frequently skewed away from older people with frailty and toward single-system conditions of young and middle-aged people [2]. Health and social care systems organized in this way might be considered as inherently ageist. This view is supported by surveys of clinicians, managers and older people [2].

In secondary care, sub-optimal care processes and hospital environments are evidenced by high rates of unintended harms such as in-patient falls and delirium. The failure to design health care systems to meet the needs of frail older people holds true even in primary care, which is traditionally considered to offer a more person-centered, holistic approach because decision support tools are largely designed for single long-term conditions. This approach works well for people of any age who have a single condition but does not work well for people with frailty.

Internationally, health care systems need to be reconfigured to meet the needs of older people with frailty. Integrated pathways are required to coordinate the care of older people with frailty, from primary care, to pre-hospital care, to the emergency department (ED), through secondary care and intermediate care to home. Well-designed pathways of care should also integrate social services and the third sector to ensure that the care needs of older people are fully met and to help to direct older people with frailty to appropriate services.

Integrated Care

Integrated care is an approach that seeks to improve the quality of care for individual patients, service users and carers by ensuring that services are well coordinated around their needs [4]. Many definitions of integrated care have been developed, but a unifying view has been proposed by an alliance of over one hundred nongovernmental organizations that represent service users in the UK (National Voices). The definition is laudably simple: 'Care that is person-centred and co-ordinated'. Three levels of integration have been described: macro (between organizations), meso (within organizations) and micro (individual care processes). Although the integration research literature has largely been predicated on the needs of people with multiple long-term conditions, all three levels of integration apply equally well to older people with frailty. This is because people with frailty frequently need to move between services and organizations and thus are particularly susceptible to the effects of the multiple assessments, delays and simple abandonment that are the characteristics of poor integration. Integrated care is achieved successfully only when the user's perspective is the organizing principle of service delivery [4]. Success requires overcoming barriers between primary and secondary care, physical and mental health, and health and social care to ensure that high-quality care is provided.

Successful models of integrated care that deliver improved quality of care for frail older people, with better outcomes and lower costs, have been identified internationally [4–6]. A range of lessons has been identified to guide the establishment of integrated care systems (table 1) [7]. Key themes that characterize successful systems include robust primary care teams at the center of the delivery system; information as a platform for guiding improvement, including electronic clinical information systems; and an approach that builds from the bottom up as well as from the top down,

Table 1. Important lessons about what is required at the local level to develop integrated care pathways

(1)	Find a common cause with partners and be prepared to share sovereignty
(2)	Develop a shared narrative to explain why integrated care matters
(3)	Develop a persuasive vision to describe what integrated care will achieve
(4)	Establish shared leadership
(5)	Create time and space to develop understanding and new ways of working
(6)	Identify services and user groups for which the potential benefits from integrated care are greatest
(7)	Build integrated care from the bottom up as well as from the top down
(8)	Pool resources to enable commissioners and integrated teams to use resources flexibly
(9)	Innovate in the use of commissioning, contracting and payment mechanisms and use of the independent sector
(10)	Recognize that there is no 'best way' of integrated care
(11)	Support and empower users to take more control over their health and wellbeing
(12)	Share information about users with the support of appropriate information governance
(13)	Use the workforce effectively and be open to innovations in the skill mix and staff substitution
(14)	Set specific objectives and measure and evaluate progress toward these objectives
(15)	Be realistic about the costs of integrated care
(16)	Act on all of these lessons together as part of a coherent strategy

including a single point of access and a single assessment process [5, 7]. One important guiding principle of integrated care is that there must be consideration of initial cost outlays for staff and support systems, new service funding and start-up costs before longer-term savings are realized [8].

Frailty Identification as a Guide for Integrated Care

A key principle of integrated care is to identify services and user groups for which the potential benefits from an integrated approach are greatest. There are several possible approaches that are relevant to people with frailty.

Risk Stratification

Risk stratification is a familiar concept in clinical medicine that is used to identify subgroups of patients with an index disease who have distinctive characteristics that impact either the outcomes of the underlying disease or the benefit/harm ratio of an intended treatment. Examples include selection of patients for cardiovascular prevention treatments or the staging process commonly applied for cancer treatments. Risk stratification is applied slightly differently in the situation of frailty; it is essentially used to distinguish older people who are frail (or degrees of frailty) from people who are not frail. In a sense, this forms a 'diagnosis' of frailty, but current clinically available tools lack the relevant level of specificity required for accurate clinical diagnosis. Some approaches to the identification of frailty, and particularly the generation of a frailty index score based on the cumulative deficit approach (Chapters 6 and 7), hold promise for identification and severity grading of frailty. If this is in fact the case, frailty diagnosis and risk stratification will become the same process.

Three broad methods for stratifying risk in older people in different health care environments are available: an age-based approach, use of validated risk stratification tools and an approach based on identification of frailty.

Age-Based Approach

The most straightforward method of risk stratification for older people is on the basis of age. Aging is a continuous life-course process. There is no biological rationale to distinguish the 'over 65s' from the 'under 65s'. This distinction, although commonly made, is sociological and relates to choices taken by developed countries in constructing employment and social care policies. Unfortunately, distinguishing on the basis of age, or ageism, has been common in health and social care. This might be acceptable if the outcomes of treating older people were inferior to those of treating younger people, but there is now considerable evidence that this is not so, with the proviso that groups with similar physiological function are compared.

Despite these reservations, age-defined separation for acute secondary care services has attracted some interest because 'old-older' people who need emergency care in the hospital are more likely to be frail. Hence, old-age cutoffs have been a popular approach to organize the separation of acutely ill older people between acute internal medicine and geriatric medicine services. This is referred to as an age-related geriatric service, and the main benefit of this approach is that it is a simple, quick and unambiguous method to stream patients at point of entry into acute care. However, it is undoubtedly crude, with proportions of fit and frail patients misplaced in both departments.

Age-defined cutoffs are also commonly used in primary care, such as for screening programs. However, the fitness spectrum of such age-defined populations is considerable, such that some included people will be unsuitable for intervention and some excluded people will be biologically fit for their years and potentially denied beneficial interventions. These types of age-defined clinical decisions sustain or propagate ageism within a health service because they provide an official justification for health care selection based on age and not on need.

Risk Stratification Tools

Several validated tools have been developed to identify and stratify people at increased risk of adverse outcomes. Examples of tools based on predictive modeling techniques include the Combined Predictive Model [9], the Patients at Risk of Rehospitalisation tool [9] and the Johns Hopkins Adjusted Clinical Groups model [10]. These tools usually use data on service use during the preceding 12 months to predict service use over the forthcoming 12 months. The tools are very heavily weighted toward predicting secondary care utilization (the main cost driver), and therefore, they try to predict a relatively rare event, i.e. hospital admissions within the source population. The precision is modest, and typically only around 1/3 of predicted 'high-risk' patients subsequently appear high risk [11]. Additionally, because these tools are rather crude, they often identify high resource users who are outside the target population, such as younger people with rare conditions, maternity cases and active cancer patients. Moreover, because these tools focus on long-term conditions, people with frailty but no long-term condition may be missed.

Although used commonly in Europe and North America, evidence for successful interventions based on risk stratification is lacking, particularly for interventions in older people, and expectations of what can be achieved through the use of risk stratification tools may be overly optimistic [12].

Routine Identification of Frailty

To facilitate the provision of goal-directed, holistic, evidence-based care, a 2013 international consensus report recommended the routine identification of frailty in people aged 70 years and over [13]. The current reference standard for identifying frailty in clinical care is comprehensive geriatric assessment (CGA) [3]. CGA has been central to good practice in elderly care medicine since the inception of specialist services for older people. It involves systems of care that can coordinate inputs from several professional disciplines. The process is effective both in identifying older people with frailty and in improving their outcomes, with the proviso that the assessment is linked to targeted intervention [14]. The main limitation of CGA is that it is a resource-intensive process in terms of both the time and the personnel required. The use of simple instruments for identifying frailty as part of routine care has been actively pursued. Additionally, the utility of existing clinical datasets to identify frailty, especially in primary care, is particularly attractive.

Simple Instruments and Questionnaires for Identifying Frailty

A range of simple instruments to identify frailty are available, but there is considerable variability in diagnostic accuracy. Table 2 summarizes the performance of a range of simple instruments to identify frailty compared to a reference-standard phenotype model. Slow gait speed appears to be the most accurate indicator for identifying frailty when compared to other simple metrics. A gait speed less than 0.8 m/s has good sensitivity (0.99) and reasonable specificity (0.64) when compared to a reference-standard phenotype model, and its measurement could be a useful test that can be performed in a range of settings to identify frailty. The presence of slow gait speed could be used to help to guide the delivery of interventions to improve outcomes and to help to inform the selection of older people for treatment with medications and invasive procedures. However, the relatively high proportion of false-positive results means that only around one in four people identified will be frail compared to a reference standard.

Table 2. Diagnostic accuracy of simple instruments for identifying frailty

Test (units)	Cutoff	Reference standard	Sensitivity	Specificity	Positive predictive value	Negative predictive value	Likelihood ratio (positive)	Likelihood ratio (negative)
Gait speed (over 75 years) (m/s)	<0.7	Phenotype model	0.92	0.69	0.41	0.97	2.98	0.10
Gait speed (over 75 years) (m/s)	<0.8	Phenotype model	0.99	0.52	0.33	0.99	2.09	0.01
Gait speed (over 75 years) (m/s)	<0.9	Phenotype model	1.00	0.44	0.30	1.00	1.78	0.00
Gait speed (m/s)	<0.7	Phenotype model	0.93	0.77	0.35	0.98	4.19	0.09
Gait speed (m/s)	<0.8	Phenotype model	0.99	0.64	0.26	0.99	2.80	0.01
Gait speed (m/s)	<0.9	Phenotype model	1.00	0.56	0.22	1.00	2.28	0.00
PRISMA 7	>3	Phenotype model	0.83	0.83	0.40	0.97	5.00	0.20
Timed up-and-go test (s)	>10	Phenotype model	0.93	0.62	0.16	0.99	2.43	0.11
Timed up-and-go test (s)	>20	Phenotype model	0.06	1.00	1.00	0.96	N/A	0.94
Self-reported health	<6	Phenotype model	0.83	0.72	0.29	0.97	3.00	0.23
GP assessment	Yes/no	Phenotype model	0.67	0.76	0.28	0.94	2.86	0.43
Polypharmacy	>5 medications	Phenotype model	0.67	0.72	0.24	0.94	2.40	0.46
Groningen frailty indicator	>4	Phenotype model	0.58	0.72	0.22	0.93	2.10	0.58

Gait speed is usually measured in m/s and has been recorded over distances ranging from 2.4 to 6 m in research studies.
The PRISMA 7 tool is a seven-item questionnaire for identifying disability that has been used in frailty studies and is suitable for postal completion. A score of ≥3 is considered to indicate frailty.
The timed up-and-go test measures, in seconds, the time taken to stand up from a standard chair, walk a distance of 3 m, turn, walk back to the chair and sit down.
Self-rated health was assessed with the question 'How would you rate your health on a scale of 0--10?'. A cut-off of ≤6 was used to define frailty.
The clinical judgment of a general practitioner (GP) involves a GP's clinical assessment and categorization as frail or not frail.
Polypharmacy is defined as the prescription of five or more medications.

Identification of Frailty Using Routinely Collected Primary Care Data

The Rockwood frailty index identifies frailty on the basis of the accumulation of a range of deficits, which are multiple patient characteristics, including clinical signs, symptoms and disease states [15]. Electronic health records use clinical codes to categorize and log multiple patient characteristics, including symptoms, signs, laboratory test results, diseases, disabilities and information about social circumstances. These records therefore provide a potentially simple yet powerful mechanism for identifying cumulative deficits to recognize and characterize frailty as part of routine care. Identification of frail older people using routinely collected data from electronic primary care database records would have considerable clinical merit, as it would be the basis for a paradigm shift in the care of frail older people toward more appropriate goal-directed care. Essentially, it would open up frailty management to the same opportunities afforded to other long-term conditions: that is, case finding, individualized care planning and multidisciplinary team reviews. The care content would be centered around promoting exercise, medication reviews, social networks, home adaptations, carer support and nutritional support. These care components, targeted at the modifiable aspects of frailty, are currently delivered sporadically rather than systematically. A validated primary care electronic frailty index would promote a shift from the currently prevalent reactive approach to frailty to a more proactive primary care model. Additionally, as the data are collected routinely, there would be no resource implications involved in generating a frailty index using electronic health records. Research has shown that this approach is feasible, although it is dependent on the quality of coded data [16].

Potential Benefits of Routine Frailty Identification in Different Settings

Routine identification of frailty would have considerable practical benefits, including the delivery of evidence-based interventions to improve outcomes and to direct improved integrated pathways of care. The benefits would potentially be applicable in a range of health and social care settings and support better care for individuals, better health for populations and lower costs.

Primary Care
Practical Benefits
Frail older people, and particularly those with cognitive impairment, need more time for the provision and assimilation of information, especially in clinical settings. They are likely to have complex care needs with multiple, interacting clinical problems. The routine identification of frailty could have simple, practical benefits, such as an increase in the length of time for routine primary care consultations.

Medication Review
Certain medications are associated with adverse outcomes in frail older people and should be avoided where possible (e.g. tricyclic antidepressants in dementia, long-acting benzodiazepines, long-acting sulfonylureas). Conversely, some medications are inappropriately omitted (e.g. angiotensin-converting enzyme inhibitors in chronic heart failure, proton pump inhibitors in severe gastro-esophageal reflux disease, antihypertensive treatments). Screening tools to detect potentially inappropriate medications and potential prescribing omissions for frail older people include the Beers criteria [17] and the STOPP/START checklist [18]. Routine identification of frailty would enable targeted evidence-based medication reviews in primary care that are based on these validated screening tools.

Provision of Evidence-Based Interventions
There is emerging evidence that targeted home-based or group-based exercise interventions may improve outcomes for frail older people, but further research is required to determine whether equivalent benefit is achieved across the frailty spectrum [19, 20]. There is emerging evidence that nutritional supplementation for those with evidence of undernutrition and that vitamin D supplements for those who are deficient may improve outcomes [13]. The identification of frailty as part of routine care would enable the selection of patients for these interventions.

Provision of Goal-Oriented Patient Care

To date, measurement of quality of care has usually focused on preventive and disease-specific care processes. Similarly, outcome measurement has typically addressed disease-specific short- and long-term indicators [21]. Disease-specific processes and outcomes are less relevant for older people with frailty, who frequently have multiple co-existing conditions and different personal priorities. An alternative approach to providing better care for older people with frailty is to identify a patient's individual health goals across a range of dimensions [21]. For example, a frail older person with hypertension, heart failure and diabetes may not see traditional outcomes of disease activity, such as blood pressure or glycated hemoglobin control, as relevant. Instead, a more meaningful, goal-oriented outcome may be to get out of a chair and walk to the toilet independently, without fear of dizziness or falling. Achieving this outcome is the purpose of the three stages of care planning [22].

Under the guidance of a person trained in care planning, the patient is encouraged to describe their 'narrative'. This is an important component, as it frames the patient's objectives in their own terms and promotes a strong therapeutic relationship between the patient and the care planner [22]. A period of reflection should then take place before the final stage of agreeing on the care plan. Correctly conducted, care planning results in profound patient engagement and highly individualized care plans that can embed preventative care strategies. Time and skill are required for successful completion. The National Health Service in England has signaled the critical role of care planning for 'vulnerable' people (this is a broad population group that includes people with frailty) and is specifically reorganizing primary care to incorporate this approach.

A goal-oriented approach has a number of advantages over the conventional approach and may enable a sense of greater control and greater ability to self-manage multiple, interacting conditions. Discussions are patient centered and are structured around individually desired health states. A focus on outcomes that span conditions and alignment toward common goals simplifies decision making for frail older people. Articulation of the relative importance and prioritization of health states is encouraged. Agreed-on steps can be taken to achieve these goals and monitor progress toward achievement.

A goal-oriented approach to the care of frail older people could enable effective shared decision making to identify the treatment strategies that are most likely to achieve patient-prioritized outcomes. Goal-oriented care for frail older people could facilitate a more holistic approach that values quality of life above the traditional, less meaningful disease centered approach to care. By identifying outcomes that are patient focused and meaningful, a goal-oriented approach would potentially have the additional benefit of improving the self-management of multiple, interacting conditions by older people with frailty.

Palliative Care
Frailty has been identified as the most common condition leading to death in community-dwelling older people [23]. However, it is not currently usual practice to begin advance care planning or to discuss end-of-life care for people with severe frailty in a timely way, which more often takes place for people with, for example, severe heart failure or terminal cancer. Identification and severity grading of frailty would enable appropriate discussions of advanced care planning, including planning the involvement of palliative care services for those with advanced frailty who are nearing the end of life.

Pre-Hospital Care
Although emergency medical service providers are well placed to identify unmet needs among frail older people, there is a paucity of research on pre-hospital care interventions [24]. One trial of a referral service for older people who call an ambulance after a fall but who are not taken to the hospital reported reduced rates of falls and improved clinical outcomes [25]. Routine identification of frailty may help to guide the development of pre-hospital care pathways for frail older people.

Emergency Department and Acute Medical Unit
Older people with frailty who are discharged from the ED are at greater risk of adverse outcomes, including subsequent hospitalization, care home admission and death [26]. Recognition that improved pathways of care are required for older people with frailty who visit EDs has led to the development of novel services. Interface geriatrics is the concept of rapid assessment, treatment and discharge for older people in crisis who visit an ED or acute medical unit. This concept usually incorporates the principle of 'discharge to assess', which is based on the premise that the unfamiliar environment of a hospital is a poor location to assess the capabilities of an older person with frailty. In 2011, a systematic review identified no clear evidence that the interface geriatrics model of care improves outcomes, including mortality, readmissions and long-term care admission, although the conclusions were limited by the very small number (n = 5) of included trials [27]. More recent evidence has demonstrated that the development of an emergency frailty unit in the ED may be associated with increased discharge rates and reduced readmissions [28]. Additionally, there is evidence that the establishment of an acute frailty admission unit that incorporates a discharge-to-assess model of care can significantly reduce the length of hospital stay with an associated reduction in mortality, without the need for extra hospital resources [29].

Acute Medical Care
Older people with frailty who receive inpatient comprehensive geriatric assessment in specialist elderly care wards are more likely to return home, are less likely to have cognitive or functional decline and have lower inpatient mortality rates than those who receive care in general medical wards [30]. Although this is the usual model of care in

some countries, including the UK, it is not an international standard. Geriatrician-led, ward-based, specialist elderly care should become the international standard of care for frail older people, and routine identification of frailty could help to guide the triage of older people to specialist elderly care wards.

Surgical Care

Older patients with fragility fractures in orthopedic wards are usually frail and often have complex comorbidity, cognitive impairment and a risk of developing delirium [31]. This has led to the establishment of the orthogeriatric model of care, in which the role of the orthogeriatrician is to address the complex needs of frail older people to ensure that they receive the same high standards of care that are attained on specialist elderly care wards. In the UK, specialist orthogeriatrician assessment is the usual model of care and is part of the UK hip fracture best practice tariff, which is a financial incentive to deliver high-quality care.

Frail older people are at greater risk of adverse outcomes following surgery, including post-operative complications, mortality, length of stay and discharge to long-term care residence [32]. Specialist assessment of frail older people at risk of adverse surgical outcomes is associated with improved outcomes, including lower rates of delirium, pressure sores and immobility [33]. The routine identification of frailty would help to guide the selection and pre-operative care of frail older people undergoing surgery.

Intermediate Care Services

There has been sustained international interest in developing novel services for older people in the virtual space between primary and secondary care. The main stimulus has been the steady rise in emergency admissions of older people against a backdrop of declining bed numbers. These competing trends have been resolved by significant reductions in length of stay, but at the potential expense of many older people leaving the hospital while incompletely recovered.

Conventional community services provide care support but aim to maintain, and not improve, function. The generic term 'intermediate care' has been used to describe these services, which essentially provide community-based support and rehabilitation care. Confusion has occurred because of the apparently disparate range of service models and the associated nomenclature (e.g. crisis/rapid response teams, virtual wards, early discharge services, re-ablement services). It is easier to understand that there is bed-based intermediate care (e.g. community hospitals) and home-based intermediate care (e.g. hospital-at-home) and that both types may have the separate functions of 'step-up' care (admission avoidance) and 'step-down' care (early discharge). The evidence base for intermediate care services is patchy. There is reasonable effectiveness evidence for community hospitals and hospital-at-home (for chronic obstructive pulmonary disease and stroke, and less so for older people with frailty), possible increased harms of nurse-led units and expensive care for care home-based rehabilitation [34].

Social Services
Older people with frailty are the main users of adult social care services in developed countries [2]. Routine identification of frailty would facilitate the direction of frail older people to appropriate services and would help to guide pathways of care.

Hospitalized frail older people who have recovered from their acute medical illness can spend many days or weeks in the hospital, waiting for the arrangement of social care support at home. Planning for hospital discharge should begin at admission, and methods to identify frailty as part of routine care could facilitate discharge planning by identifying those who are more likely to need increased social care or rehabilitation.

Improving the Organization of Health and Social Care for Older People with Frailty

The priorities of care for older people with frailty should be to prevent acute health crises, to manage exacerbations of chronic disease and to support independent living at home. This requires collaboration between health and social care providers to develop integrated care pathways that deliver a comprehensive set of services. Pathways should span primary and secondary care, intermediate care and social services.

Older people with frailty, and particularly those with cognitive impairment and dementia, are at their most vulnerable when they present to the hospital with an acute illness. The development of integrated care pathways for frailty should ensure that systems exist for sharing information at critical points in the patient's journey.

Detection of frailty should be an essential part of assessment of older people. Failure to detect frailty potentially exposes patients to interventions that may not be beneficial and that indeed could be harmful. Conversely, excluding fit older people, on the basis of age alone, from interventions from which they may benefit is unacceptable [3]. Identification of slow gait speed is a simple test that can be performed in a range of locations to detect frailty and could be used to guide the delivery of evidence-based care to frail older people. However, this measurement has staff resource implications and may be inaccurate. The identification of frailty using existing clinical data to construct a frailty index on the basis of the cumulative deficit model is attractive. This approach would enable positive identification and severity grading of frailty. This would have considerable clinical merit because it would be the basis for a paradigm shift in the care of frail older people toward a more goal-directed model of care.

References

1 Rockwood K, Hubbard R: Frailty and the geriatrician. Age Ageing 2004;33:429–430.
2 Oliver D: Age based discrimination in health and social care services. BMJ 2009;339:b3400.
3 Clegg A, Young J, Iliffe S, Olde Rikkert M, Rockwood K: Frailty in elderly people. Lancet 2013;381:752–762.

4 Goodwin N, Smith J, Davies A, Perry C, Rosen R, Dixon A, Dixon J, Ham C: Integrated Care for Patients and Populations: Improved Outcomes by Working Together. London, The King's Fund, 2012.
5 Baker GR, Denis J-L: A Comparative Study of Three Transformative Healthcare Systems: Lessons for Canada. Ottawa, Canadian Health Services Research Foundation, 2011.
6 Ashton CM, Souchek J, Petersen NJ, Menke TJ, Collins TC, Kizer KW, Wright SM, Wray NP: Hospital use and survival among Veterans Affairs beneficiaries. N Engl J Med 2003;349:1637–1646.
7 Ham C, Walsh N: Making Integrated Care Happen at Scale and Pace. London, The King's Fund, 2013.
8 Leutz W: Five laws for integrating medical and social services: lessons from the United States and the United Kingdom. Millbank Quarterly 1999;77:77–110.
9 Georghiou T: Predictive Risk and Health Care: An Overview. London, Nuffield Trust, 2011.
10 Weiner JP, Starfield BH, Steinwachs DM, Mumford LM: Development and application of a population-oriented measure of ambulatory care case-mix. Med Care 1991;29:452–472.
11 Hoch I, Heymann A, Karpati T, Valinsky L: C-C2-02: Validation and uses of the ACG-DX predictive modeling and risk adjustment tool in an Israeli HMO. Clin Med Res 2010;8:51–52.
12 Roland M, Abel G: Reducing emergency admissions: are we on the right track? BMJ 2012;345:e6017.
13 Morley JE, Vellas B, van Kan GA, Anker SD, Bauer JM, Bernabei R, Cesari M, Chumlea WC, Doehner W, Evans J, Fried LP, Guralnik JM, Katz PR, Malmstrom TK, McCarter RJ, Gutierrez Robledo LM, Rockwood K, von Haehling S, Vandewoude MF, Walston J: Frailty consensus: a call to action. J Am Med Dir Assoc 2013;14:392–397.
14 Beswick AD, Rees K, Dieppe P, Ayis S, Gooberman-Hill R, Horwood J, Ebrahim S: Complex interventions to improve physical function and maintain independent living in elderly people: a systematic review and meta-analysis. Lancet 2008;371:725–735.
15 Mitnitski AB, Mogilner AJ, Rockwood K: Accumulation of deficits as a proxy measure of aging. ScientificWorldJournal 2001;1:323–336.
16 Drubbel I, de Wit NJ, Bleijenberg N, Eijkemans RJ, Schuurmans MJ, Numans ME: Prediction of adverse health outcomes in older people using a frailty index based on routine primary care data. J Gerontol A Biol Sci Med Sci 2012;68:301–308.
17 Fick DM, Cooper JW, Wade WE, Waller JL, Maclean JR, Beers MH: Updating the Beers criteria for potentially inappropriate medication use in older adults: results of a US consensus panel of experts. Arch Intern Med 2003;163:2716–2724.
18 Ryan C, O'Mahony D, Kennedy J, Weedle P, Byrne S: Potentially inappropriate prescribing in an Irish elderly population in primary care. Br J Clin Pharmacol 2009;68:936–947.
19 Clegg A, Barber S, Young J, Forster A, Iliffe S: Do home-based exercise interventions improve outcomes for frail older people? Findings from a systematic review. Rev Clin Gerontol 2012;22:68–78.
20 Theou O, Stathokostas L, Roland KP, Jakobi JM, Patterson C, Vandervoort AA, Jones GR: The effectiveness of exercise interventions for the management of frailty: a systematic review. J Aging Res 2011;2011: 569194.
21 Reuben DB, Tinetti ME: Goal-oriented patient care–an alternative health outcomes paradigm. N Engl J Med 2012;366:777–779.
22 Mathers N, Roberts S, Hodkinson I, Karet B: Care Planning: Improving the Lives of People with Long Term Conditions. London, Royal College of General Practitioners, 2011.
23 Gill TM, Gahbauer EA, Han L, Allore HG: Trajectories of disability in the last year of life. N Engl J Med 2010;362:1173–1180.
24 Goldstein JP, Andrew MK, Travers A: Frailty in older adults using pre-hospital care and the emergency department: a narrative review. Can Geriatr J 2012; 15:16–22.
25 Logan PA, Coupland CA, Gladman JR, Sahota O, Stoner-Hobbs V, Robertson K, Tomlinson V, Ward M, Sach T, Avery AJ: Community falls prevention for people who call an emergency ambulance after a fall: randomised controlled trial. BMJ 2010;340: c2102.
26 Hastings SN, Purser JL, Johnson KS, Sloane RJ, Whitson HE: Frailty predicts some but not all adverse outcomes in older adults discharged from the emergency department. J Am Geriatr Soc 2008;56: 1651–1657.
27 Conroy SP, Stevens T, Parker SG, Gladman JR: A systematic review of comprehensive geriatric assessment to improve outcomes for frail older people being rapidly discharged from acute hospital: 'interface geriatrics'. Age Ageing 2011;40:436–443.
28 Conroy SP, Ansari K, Williams M, Laithwaite E, Teasdale B, Dawson J, Mason S, Banerjee J: A controlled evaluation of comprehensive geriatric assessment in the emergency department: the 'Emergency Frailty Unit'. Age Ageing 2014;43:109–114.
29 Silvester K, Mohammed M, Harriman P, Girolami A, Downes T: Timely care for frail older people referred to hospital improves efficiency and reduces mortality without the need for extra resources. Age Ageing 2014;43:472–477.

30 Ellis G, Whitehead MA, Robinson D, O'Neill D, Langhorne P: Comprehensive geriatric assessment for older adults admitted to hospital: meta-analysis of randomised controlled trials. BMJ 2011;343: d6553.
31 Marcantonio ER, Flacker JM, Wright RJ, Resnick NM: Reducing delirium after hip fracture: a randomized trial. J Am Geriatr Soc 2001;49:516–522.
32 Lacas A, Rockwood K: Frailty in primary care: a review of its conceptualization and implications for practice. BMC Med 2012;10:4.
33 Harari D, Hopper A, Dhesi J, Babic-Illman G, Lockwood L, Martin F: Proactive care of older people undergoing surgery ('POPS'): designing, embedding, evaluating and funding a comprehensive geriatric assessment service for older elective surgical patients. Age Ageing 2007;36:190–196.
34 Young J: The development of intermediate care services in England. Arch Gerontol Geriatr 2009; 49(suppl 2):S21–S25.

Dr. Andrew Clegg
Academic Unit of Elderly Care and Rehabilitation, University of Leeds
Temple Bank House, Bradford Teaching Hospitals NHS Foundation Trust
Duckworth Lane
Bradford BD9 6RJ (UK)
E-Mail a.p.clegg@leeds.ac.uk

Theou O, Rockwood K (eds): Frailty in Aging. Biological, Clinical and Social Implications.
Interdiscipl Top Gerontol Geriatr. Basel, Karger, 2015, vol 41, pp 174–185 (DOI: 10.1159/000381235)

Frailty's Place in Ethics and Law: Some Thoughts on Equality and Autonomy and on Limits and Possibilities for Aging Citizens

Mary McNally[a] · William Lahey[b]

[a]Faculties of Dentistry and Medicine and [b]Schulich School of Law and School of Health Administration, Dalhousie University, Halifax, N.S., Canada

Abstract

Consideration of ethical and legal themes relating to frailty must engage with the concern that frailty is a pejorative concept that validates and reinforces the disadvantage and vulnerability of aging adults. In this chapter, we consider whether a greater focus on frailty may indeed be part of the solution to the disadvantages that aging adults face in achieving equality and maintaining their autonomy within systems that have used their frailty to deny them equality and autonomy. First, by examining equality both as an ethical norm and as a requirement for protections against discrimination, we raise questions about the grounds on which health providers and health systems can be required to give equal concern and respect to the needs of frail older persons. Second, we explore autonomy and identify the tension between meaningful self-determination and prevailing ethical and legal norms associated with informed choice. Third, we argue that a proper understanding of frailty is essential within both of these themes; it respects equality by enabling health providers and systems to identify and address the distinct care needs of aging adults and helps to align informed choice theory with appropriate processes for decision-making about those needs.

The purpose of this chapter is to identify known ethical and legal themes in health care within the framework of frailty and to identify related unresolved questions. Given that the frailty epidemic is an emerging phenomenon, ethical/legal questions with specific relevance to those who are frail remain insufficiently examined. Even less examined is the extent to which use of 'frailty' as a pejorative label, predisposing older adults to paternalism, negative stereotypes and discrimination [1], can coexist and be reconciled with the unifying and advancing understanding of frailty as a complex health syndrome that is central to providing appropriate care and support to millions of aging people.

To focus this discussion, we have considered frailty as a vulnerable state in order to identify and explore two key areas where ethics and law clearly intersect: (1) equality, understood both as a relevant ethical norm and as a requirement for legal protections against discrimination when equality is denied, ignored or simply not recognized, and (2) autonomy and the tension that arises between meaningful self-determination in health care and the legally mandated and prevailing ethical norms associated with 'informed choice'.

Equality

One of the universal functions of equality law is to protect people against discrimination based on age and other personal characteristics. Older people unquestionably and routinely face discrimination because of their age, including in the health care system [2–4]. Often, age-based discrimination intersects with other prohibited grounds of discrimination, including disability, sex (or gender), race, national or ethnic origin, aboriginal status, religion, and sexual orientation [4].

At the center of their vulnerability to discrimination is the frequency with which older persons are treated on the basis of stereotypes or in ways that reinforce stereotypes. A pervasive element of these stereotypes is the assumption that older persons are, by virtue of being old, also frail, weak, needy, and lacking or diminished in capacity or potential. By extension, they are understood to require less or be less deserving of goods, services, benefits and opportunities than others. This broader and intrinsic devaluation of old age by society at large is commonly understood as 'ageism' [5]. Of significance to this chapter is that evolving conceptions of ageism over the last several decades suggest that ageism, understood historically to focus on all older adults, has been more recently reserved for application to frail and disabled elders. Moreover, issues of ageism have moved from primarily moral discussions to the arena of legal obligation through legislative enactments focused on age discrimination [5].

In this context, the concern is that characterizing frailty as a biophysical attribute and using it as the basis for clinical decision-making provides validation and objectivity to ageism [6]. Within health care, for example, a diagnosis of relative frailty may be applied deterministically to provide justification for limiting, withholding or denying certain kinds of care and for exposing older persons to greater loss of their autonomy in clinical decision-making than they may already typically face. More broadly, a diagnosis of 'being frail' could expose diagnosed persons to broader and perhaps more intractable discrimination, beyond the health and social care systems in their homes, social networks and communities.

In broad strokes, the concern is that the 'medicalization' of frailty will reinforce the socially constructed nature of ageism inside and outside health care [7]. This concern runs in the same direction as critiques of a medicalized understanding of disability and the role that it can play in preventing attention to the social construction of disability and legitimizing clinical approaches that can reinforce stereotypes and undermine autonomy by, for example, subsuming neurological differences within the concept of mental illness [8–10].

Conversely, the premise of numerous chapters in this book is that frailty must be understood and taken into account because frailty – or its absence – is critical to understanding care that benefits older adults [11]. In this view, clarifying a person's place on a 'frailty spectrum' helps to ensure that older persons are informed, diagnosed and treated in 'correspondence' with their actual 'needs, circumstances and capacities', the concept used in Canadian constitutional law to distinguish between valid differentiations on the basis of age (or other grounds of discrimination) and differentiations that stereotype [12]. In health care, differentiating between the needs of patients based on their relative frailty may avoid differentiation on the basis of age and mitigate age-based discrimination. In the United Kingdom, where denial of care based on age alone is explicitly prohibited, it is argued that health care must come to terms with frailty to prevent efforts to address the different and varied needs of older patients from being understood and characterized as age discrimination [13]. Moreover, since substantive equality means affirmative action in response to disadvantage as well as avoidance of negative discrimination, true equality requires more than avoidance of the pejorative connotation of frailty. It also requires recognition, understanding and responsiveness to frailty. As argued in the introductory chapter of this book, there is nothing about frailty that is made better by not talking about it.

Equality means more than protection from discrimination. It can be seen as a fundamental aim or consequence of justice and is understood as the fair, equitable and appropriate treatment owed to persons (e.g. equal political rights and access to equal public services such as health care) [14]. Whether or not there is an enforceable legal right to this broader equality, it operates as an ethical and political norm [14, 15] and calls on governments and health care systems to ensure a defensible measure of equality of access to needed care, including for vulnerable populations [16]. Older adults, because of the equal value of the lives that they have to live, deserve responsive and proportionate attention to their particular health care needs [17]. In the language of Canadian equality law, equality of older persons requires that their needs be given 'equal concern and respect' in health care, as elsewhere [18]. The feasibility of these commitments is typically questioned out of fear that the consumption of health care by the 'grey tsunami' will make health care systems socially unaffordable and unable to meet the needs of other demographics. The response from an equality perspective often includes a mounting of the barricades against any hint of age-based rationing.

Polarized debate overlooks the evidence suggesting that population aging plays a small part in the growth of health care spending [19, 20]. What does matter is how the health care system responds to need; here, it is relevant that health systems tend to provide older adults with too much or too little care [21]. On the one hand, they excel at providing conventional illness-specific interventions, with insufficient regard for the higher risk and the lower potential benefits for older persons. On the other hand, they struggle to provide older adults with integrated and continuous programs of care and chronic disease management that are responsive to older adults' complex needs. The reconfiguration required is complex. It goes well beyond what can be accomplished by health care practitioners. Broad changes to how resources are allocated at every scale of decision-making; how providers are educated, compensated and supported in their roles; how aging adults and their families are supported; and how systems of health and social care designed to fix or ameliorate specific problems are needed to understand and address a totality of continuing, escalating and interacting health and social needs.

Nevertheless, by systematically and comprehensively seeking a better understanding of frailty and its significance to the real needs of patients, health care practitioners play an influential role in establishing defensible clinical approaches to care as well as requisite accompanying rehabilitative and social supports. A change in health care practice can contribute to a foundation on which to reconfigure broader system changes.

Those changes must be pursued with due concern for how fair health care decisions are made in the face of finite resources. This is especially pertinent for those older adults who are especially vulnerable to ageism-based discrimination. A lack of clarity about the needs, circumstances and capacity of older adults or the presence of idiosyncratic care practices increase the possibility that the decisions will be made through legal channels that tend to push toward binary choices, rather than through reflective deliberation by the broad spectrum of stakeholders who should be influencing health care and health policy. A useful alternative framework, and one that is gaining international attention as a dominant decision-making paradigm in other realms of health care [22], is the 'accountability for reasonableness framework' conceptualized by Daniels and Sabin [16]. In this view, in order to achieve fair and justifiable limits for health care spending, fair processes for priority setting are a necessary condition for establishing and sustaining the legitimacy of system-wide decisions [16, 23]. Process elements that could contribute to legitimate decision-making relevant to frailty include explicit priority setting, transparent deliberation, input beyond that of medical experts and outcome measures that matter to patients [16].

Autonomy and Informed Choice

A key and universal ethical principle for those who influence health care is to facilitate choices that maximize benefit and minimize harm on behalf of patients and members of the public [14]. Choices about benefits and harms must be offered with meaningful consideration for both personal autonomy and the values and preferences of those affected. 'Autonomy' refers simply to the 'rule of self', which is free from interferences and is a central value in Western health care [14, 24]. It assumes that we, as autonomous individuals, are able to act intentionally, with understanding and without controlling interferences. At the patient encounter, respect for autonomy is predominantly operationalized through care providers' obligation to enable others to act on their own understanding of their own best interest when making health care decisions [14, 24].

Whether arising from philosophical, medical or legal perspectives, this obligation translates into five commonly accepted elements of informed choice, or, in the language of law in Canada and other countries, informed consent [14, 25]. These include preconditions of patient voluntariness (an absence of coercion or undue influence); capacity (the ability to understand information relevant to a decision and to reasonably appreciate the foreseeable consequences); understanding (comprehension of all pertinent information); the disclosure element (provision of all pertinent information); and finally, authorization of a choice by the patient.

Respecting the autonomy of patients through the informed choice process is often nuanced and complicated, but it is a professional obligation that practitioners should take very seriously. Whereas informed choice provides the doorway into the patient relationship, its absence results in serious ethical and legal breaches. From an ethical perspective, this absence may be the result of paternalistic influences (possibly even motivated by good intentions and other ethical obligations such as beneficence), or worse, it may be suggestive of disregard for patients' values or rights to self-determination. Whatever the motivation, from a legal perspective, it is civilly actionable. For example, it is actionable in Canada as battery and in Australia as trespass [25, 26]. Treatment without valid informed choice can also be prosecuted criminally as assault.

Ethical and legal considerations play out in a number of ways with respect to the elements introduced above. As noted, valid informed choice implies that the choice be authorized by someone who has the capacity to make decisions based on his or her ability to understand material information as well as the foreseeable consequences of the decision. Where a patient lacks capacity, the law typically requires that informed choice be sought from a capable person who has legal authority to decide on behalf of the patient. In Canada and many other countries, patients are assumed to have capacity unless they are determined to be incapable under the applicable legal test.

Informed choice must be voluntary; duress or coercion, including undue influence by clinicians regarding what may be best for patients, is not genuine choice. It must also be authorized by a patient (or a substitute decision-maker) who has been adequately informed of the risks that are material to the choice between undergoing and not undergoing the proposed treatment or between alternative treatments. This places a duty on the treating clinician to disclose all material risks. The duty to disclose enables informed patient decision-making where bodily integrity and self-determination are at stake. In consequence, the scope of the duty is broad. Its breadth is determined by the patient's need to know, not by the views of the health care provider. Disclosure must therefore address all of the information on the likelihood of predicted clinical outcomes and the gravity of associated risks that a reasonable patient would regard as material. In addition, it must address the risks that the health care provider knows or ought to know the patient would regard as material when these are beyond or different from the risks that a reasonable patient would regard as material.

Integral to disclosure of material information is its understanding by patients. It is important to recognize that the capacity to understand information and actual understanding achieved through effective disclosure are distinct elements of informed choice. A person may indeed have the capacity or ability to understand information relevant to alternative choices but may be left without actual understanding of that information after its inadequate disclosure and explanation. For example, technical jargon or unfamiliar language may impede patients' understanding of information that is material to their choice. Actual understanding requires that information be disclosed in a manner that is meaningful to those who are making the choices. Therefore, health providers are also obliged to ensure that material information and risk associated with alternative choices are understood by patients.

When disclosure is found to be inadequate (and this includes a failure to meet the test of patient understanding) and resulting in patient harm, the responsible provider can be liable. In Canada and, similarly, in Australia, this liability would be dealt with under the law of negligence. Here, the patient must show that he or she suffered harm in consequence of the choice that he or she made and that a reasonable patient given adequate disclosure would have made a different treatment choice.

This legal and ethical framework, painted here in very broad strokes, has a range of implications for the care and treatment of those who are frail. Most obviously, like other patients, they are entitled to have the same control over their health care that informed choice is intended to give to all capable patients. Indeed, if what the authors of this book say about the importance of frailty to the clinical need and capacity of those who are relatively frail is accurate, true fidelity to the concept of informed choice and its underlying value of autonomy creates an imperative for a better understanding of frailty and its relationship to health care decision-making [15]. The alternative is decision-making that is materially uniformed. Likewise, as our knowledge of frailty and its relevance to the care and treatment of older adults expands and our ability to apply that knowledge through dependable diagnostic tools increases, it will become increasingly clear that informed decision-making by older adults requires disclosure and understanding of their relative position on the fitness-to-frailty spectrum. In other words, if the duty of disclosure is taken seriously, frailty and its relevance to specific treatment options become necessary and critical considerations for clinical decision-making.

However, a range of systemic obstacles stand in the way of providers aiming to integrate frailty into their efforts to respect the right of frail patients to fully informed choice. Here, we discuss three: the role that standards of practice can play to divert attention from choice, the relative unavailability of research evidence applicable to frail patients, and the gaps between the process and theory of informed choice and the reality of frail older adults.

For the first of these, the pressure to follow standards of practice, whether or not they reflect the best interests of frail patients, causes normalization of aggressive and life-advancing treatment alternatives for adults of advanced age. Increasingly accepted as standard practices, these treatments serve to undermine meaningful choice by mobilizing hope about interventions that are often accompanied with questionable gains while, at the same time, failing to account for risks associated with both the condition and the procedures themselves [27]. According to Shim and coworkers [27], 'understandings of the mandate to treat at ever-older ages contribute, pragmatically, to the elimination of any significant deliberation about whether or not to treat'. Instead, 'standard practice replaces choice', a danger that is reinforced by the reality that options for older adults experiencing frailty are not so clear [28]. The result can be harm to individuals who are provided treatment options without sufficient consideration of the risk arising from frailty. Coronary artery bypass surgery provides a striking example, illustrating high risks of adverse outcomes in frail patients, most of whom will either die (15%) or become catastrophically disabled (50%) following surgery [29, 30].

The second systemic barrier to integrating frailty into informed choice is the relative unavailability of research evidence that is readily applicable to frail patients. A number of earlier chapters present current best evidence associated with evaluating and managing frailty in a variety of health services and social contexts, yet it is fair to suggest that health research related to frailty is still a nascent frontier. The void in medical evidence available to adequately inform health care for those who are frail creates a conundrum, particularly for clinicians who face the legal imperative to disclose current best evidence to facilitate informed decision-making. For instance, older adults, and especially those who lack capacity, are systematically excluded from research trials; this is highly problematic, considering that older adults are known to suffer the greatest collective health burdens [31]. Health interventions to address chronic diseases in older adults are likely to have different outcomes for those who are frail versus those who are not frail [32]. Adding to this conundrum is difficulty in even advancing the research agenda to be suitably appropriate for frail older adults. Not surprisingly, comorbidity, exhaustion and respondent burden are identified as contributing to the high attrition rates of frail research participants [28].

Over the past decade, international stakeholder and large expert workgroups have examined emerging research challenges [32], attempted to address research disparities and challenged the assumption that frail older adults would not tolerate or benefit from research [28, 31, 32]. Numerous strategies to augment research validity for frail patients continue to emerge, including the development of relevant research guidelines; improvements to recruitment, such as eligibility screening, inclusion criteria, and increasing conventional sample sizes to account for attrition; and expansion of outcome measures to include proxy and quality-of-life measures in addition to objective biomedical outcomes and validation of novel secondary outcomes.

In the meantime, the need for large-scale trials and interventions that meaningfully include the needs of older adults remains urgent. Without their inclusion, current best evidence does not sufficiently reflect pertinent outcomes or risks. It follows, then, that for the purposes of informed decision-making, health outcomes associated with research interventions and trials that do not include the participation of frail older adults, or even adults with comorbidities, should only be judiciously extended to those who are frail, if indeed these outcomes are extended at all [28].

This brings us to the third systemic barrier: the gap between the logic of the process and theory of informed choice and the complex reality of the situation of frail patients. Understanding the frailty of older adults can clearly have implications for the implementation of the process of informed choice for older adults. It is well recognized that older patients are among those for whom the gap between the theory and the reality of informed choice is likely to be significant. In keeping with earlier references to ageism, frail older adults are particularly vulnerable to paternalistic health care, which assumes a diminished ability to understand and to make decisions in the face of complex information options. Taken to an extreme, these attitudes can result in mistaken conclusions about the capacity of older adults. Short of that, there is the risk that older adults will not be given a full explanation of all of the information to which they are entitled to fully assess their clinical options or adequate assistance in understanding that information.

Considering frailty as a diagnostic characterization or clinical condition could accentuate these problems by giving validation to or rationalizing the assumption that frail older adults lack the capacity to fully adhere to the concept of informed choice. This risk is even greater if the diagnostic criteria for frailty emphasize diminished autonomy (i.e. cognitive functioning or physical dependency) that is more susceptible to deterministic application. Therefore, the wider use of frailty as a diagnostic characterization will give additional urgency to implementation of the range of positive actions that can be taken to address and mitigate the challenges that older adults face in exercising the right of informed choice in substance as well as in form. One of these actions is education for providers, patients, family members, health administrators and policy-makers. Another is a more deliberate and organized approach to the wider implementation of the concept of assisted or supported decision-making for older patients [33]. Another, which is closely related, is the development and implementation of measures to improve the ways in which information is shared with and explained to older adults and to give older adults and their family members better decision-making support. Such measures would not only guard against the risk of frailty being equated with incapacity; they would also respond to the reality that the elderly frail often do have diminished ability to effectively exercise their rights precisely when the volume and complexity of information relevant to their health is likely to be high.

In this regard, taking frailty seriously as a significant variable in caring for older adults could support the call of ethicists for a reconsideration of our understanding of self-determination in health care. Given the value placed on autonomy in Western culture, it is not difficult to appreciate why self-determination is a dominant and highly privileged principle. However, recent ethics discourse suggests that autonomy, as it is traditionally understood and applied in health care, is problematic [34, 35]. Illness, by its very nature, tends to make patients dependent on the care and good will of others and reduces patients' power to exercise autonomy [34]. As a state of increased vulnerability, frailty likewise connotes dependency, a circumstance that does not lend itself to autonomous agency. Consequently, there is a need to consider a more relational conception of autonomy, one that recognizes dependency as well as the influences that exist for patients within their care relationships [35]. This may have profound implications for how we think about and operationalize informed choice in this context. At the very least, it suggests the need for expectations, institutional structures and processes that advance assisted or supported decision-making as the norm.

More, and not less, attention to frailty may be needed to close the gaps between informed choice theory and the reality for aging adults. Frailty, as explored in this book, could be the integrating concept that allows a different kind of informed choice, one that is an inclusive, comprehensive and manageable process. Currently, the theory of informed choice plays out similarly to the ways in which health care interventions are applied; choices are often offered in relation to 'one condition at a time'. Other chapters in this book attest to the importance of considering the constellation of factors that contribute simultaneously to frailty (i.e. the totality of issues), rather than incremental and discrete health care needs. Older adults are more likely to have multiple chronic conditions that call not only for specific treatment of specific illnesses by specific providers but also for the continuing management of their chronic conditions by multidisciplinary teams working throughout the subsectors of the health and social care systems.

Just as health care systems struggle to coordinate and integrate programs of care, they struggle to efficiently and effectively align these programs with the informed choice process. The result can be informed choice on aspects of care or treatment that does not account for the relationship of that care or treatment to the larger context of the patient's clinical condition or continuing program of care. The informed choice process can become a burden to patients, family members and providers, as it is applied to each and every event in the patient's course of treatment as if each were a distinct health care event, rather than part of a continuous process of care.

These dynamics may call for a reconfiguration of the informed choice process to better align it with the health condition of older adults and the health care choices that they typically face. Understanding frailty as a distinct clinical condition, as explored in this book, suggests a need for such a reconfiguration while, at the same time, providing guidance on how that might be accomplished. This understanding demonstrates that the complex and multifaceted needs of many older adults are the result not only of the onset of the multiple distinct illnesses of age but also of a common underlying condition that explains the interaction and effect of other conditions and the options for their amelioration. This understanding of frailty also provides guidance on how informed choice can be reconfigured by showing how it can be integrated and organized into programs of health and social care that have therapeutic coherence and unity based on their concern with the relative frailty of patients.

Concluding Thoughts

Consideration of ethical and legal issues relating to frailty must engage with the concern that frailty is a pejorative concept that validates and reinforces the disadvantages and vulnerability of aging adults. From this perspective, we offer a counterintuitive conclusion: that a greater focus on frailty may be part of the solution to the disadvantages that aging adults face in achieving equality and maintaining their autonomy within systems that have used their frailty to deny them equality and autonomy.

To foster equality, a properly informed and applied understanding of frailty can be one of the keys to ensuring that health and social systems not only do not use age as a reason for denying care but also are fully responsive to the distinct care needs of aging adults. In the realm of autonomy, this kind of focus on frailty can help to align informed choice process and theory with the real and typically different health and social needs of aging citizens. In both of these sentences, the operative word is 'can'. What matters is not only how we understand frailty but also how we apply that understanding to ensure that it advances equality, autonomy and justice for aging citizens.

Unanswered Questions

The chapters in this book represent insights about frailty and its management, ranging from examination of biophysical and clinical advances to considerations for primary, hospital and continuing care, and further to the complexities of organizational, policy and social contexts that influence the lived experience of those who are frail. Each of these themes has the potential to raise many important ethical and legal questions, and especially normative questions that arise when choices have to be made about what ought to happen within particular contexts and among competing values. While we chose to focus on only a couple of themes at the intersection of ethics and law, our reflections identify further key unanswered questions regarding frailty within these themes:

(1) Will the diagnosis and treatment of frailty as a distinct clinical and social condition expose older adults to discrimination on the basis of age? Will it help to protect them from age-based discrimination?

(2) Are the recognition of frailty as a distinct clinical diagnosis and the use of frailty as a basis for decision-making in health and social services likely to exacerbate or ameliorate the vulnerability of older adults?

(3) Will increased representation of frail older adults in research protocols serve to ameliorate the injustice of their current under-representation, or will it create other ethical concerns related to respecting their welfare by mitigating exposure to undue physical hardship or impositions on personal autonomy?

(4) Does a shift to new paradigms for diagnosing and managing frailty depend on a broader shift from autonomy to relational autonomy? Should it involve a parallel shift from 'substitute' to 'supported' decision-making?

(5) What changes to the legal framework for professional practice, to the organization of funding, and to the delivery of health and social services can or must be made to facilitate or enable improved diagnosis and treatment and management of frailty?

(6) How is frailty relevant to (or related to) our understanding of the capacity of older adults to make decisions for themselves? Does our evolving understanding of frailty, its dynamics and its consequences have implications for our understanding and evaluation of the capacity of older adults?

Acknowledgments

This chapter evolved from a Nova Scotia Health Research Foundation capacity-building grant. The authors gratefully acknowledge Dr. Stephen Birch for contributions to early discussions as well as research assistance from Emma Baasch, Karen MacNeil and Lyndsay Foisey.

References

1 Richardson S, Karunananthan S, Bergman H: I may be frail but i ain't no failure. Can Geriatr J 2011;14: 24–28.
2 Ontario Human Rights Commission: A Time for Action: Advancing Human Rights for Older Ontarians. Toronto, Ontario Human Rights Commission, 2001.
3 van Heuvel WJA, van Santvoort MM: Experienced discrimination amongst European old citizens. Eur J Ageing 2011;8:291–299.
4 Law Commission of Ontario: A Framework for the Law as it Affects Older Adults: Advancing Substantive Equality for Older Persons through Law, Policy and Practice. Toronto, Law Commission of Ontario, 2012.
5 Cohen ES: The complex nature of ageism: what is it? Who does it? Who perceives it? Gerontologist 2001; 41:576–577.
6 Special Senate Committee on Aging: Canada's Aging Population: Seizing the Opportunity. Ottawa, Special Senate Committee on Aging, 2009.
7 Hall M: Old age (or, do we need a critical theory of law and aging?) Windsor Review of Legal and Social Issues 2014;1.
8 Bickenbach JE, Chatterji S, Badley EM, Üstün TB: Models of disablement, universalism and the international classification of impairments, disabilities and handicaps. Soc Sci Med 1999;48:1173–1187.
9 Kaiser HA: Canadian mental health law: the slow process of redirecting the ship of state. Health Law J 2009;17:139–194.
10 Carver PJ: Mental health law in Canada; in Downie J, Caulfield T, Flood C (eds): Canadian Health Law and Policy, ed 3. Toronto, LexisNexis Canada Inc., 2007, pp 399–436.
11 Mallery LH, Moorhouse P: Respecting frailty. J Med Ethics 2011;37:126–128.
12 Law v. Canada (Minister of Employment and Immigration) 1999, 1 SCR 497.

13 Romero-Ortuno R, O'Shea D: Fitness and frailty: opposite ends of a challenging continuum! Will the end of age discrimination make frailty assessments an imperative? Age Ageing 2013;42:270–280.
14 Beauchamp TL, Childress JF: Principles of Biomedical Ethics, ed 7. New York, Oxford University Press, 2013.
15 Asada Y: Health Inequality: Morality and Measurement. Toronto, University of Toronto Press, 2007.
16 Daniels N, Sabin JE: Setting Limits Fairly: Learning to Share Resources for Health, ed 2. Oxford: Oxford University Press, 2008.
17 Giordano S: Respect for equality and the treatment of the elderly: declarations of human rights and age-based rationing. Camb Q Healthc Ethics 2005;14:83–92.
18 Alon-Shenker P: The unequal right to equality: towards a dignified lives approach to age discrimination. Can J Law Jurisprudence 2012;25:243–282.
19 Dormont B, Grignon M, Huber H: Health expenditure growth: reassessing the threat of aging. Health Econ 2006;15:947–963.
20 Canadian Institute of Health Information: Health Care in Canada, 2011: A Focus on Seniors. Ottawa, Canadian Institute for Health Information, 2011.
21 Rockwood K: An unsuitable old age: the paradoxes of elder care. CMAJ 2005;173:1500–1501.
22 Martin DK, Giacomini M, Singer P: Fairness, accountability for reasonableness, and the views of priority setting decision-makers. Health Policy 2002;61:279–290.
23 Daniels N: Accountability for reasonableness: establishing a fair process for priority setting is easier than agreeing on principles. BMJ 2000;321:1300–1301.
24 Entwistle VA, Carter SM, Cribb A, McCaffery K: Supporting patient autonomy: the importance of clinician-patient relationships. J Gen Intern Med 2010;25:741–745.
25 Peppin P: Informed consent; in Downie J, Caulfield T, Flood C (eds): Canadian Health Law and Policy, ed 4. Markham, Ontario, LexisNexis Canada Inc., 2011, pp 153–194.
26 Richards P: General principles of consent to medical treatment; in White B, McDonald F, Willmot L (eds): Health Law in Australia. Pyrmont, N.S.W., Lawbook Co./Thomson Reuters, 2010, pp 93–111.
27 Shim JK, Russ AJ, Kaufman SR: Risk, life extension and the pursuit of medical possibility. Sociol Health Illn 2006;28:479–502.
28 Ferrucci L, Guralnik JM, Studenski S, Fried LP, Cutler GB Jr, Walston JD; Interventions on Frailty Working Group: Designing randomized, controlled trials aimed at preventing or delaying functional decline and disability in frail, older persons: a consensus report. J Am Geriatr Soc 2004;52:625–634.
29 Lee DH, Buth KJ, Martin BJ, Yip AM, Hirsch GM: Frail patients are at increased risk for mortality and prolonged institutional care after cardiac surgery. Circulation 2010;121:973–978.
30 Afilalo J, Mottillo S, Eisenberg MJ, Alexander KP, Noiseux N, Perrault LP, Morin JF, Langlois Y, Ohayon SM, Monette J, Boivin JF, Shahian DM, Bergman H: Addition of frailty and disability to cardiac surgery risk scores identifies elderly patients at high risk of mortality or major morbidity. Circ Cardiovasc Qual Outcomes 2012;5:222–228.
31 Herrara AP, Snipes SA, King DW, Torres-Vigil I, Goldberg DS, Weinberg AD: Disparate inclusion of older adults in clinical trials: priorities and opportunities for policy and practice change. Am J Public Health 2010;100:S105–S112.
32 Bergman H, Ferrucci L, Guralnik J, Hogan DB, Hummel S, Karunananthan S, Wolfson C: Frailty: an emerging research and clinical paradigm – issues and controversies. J Gerontol 2007;62A:731–737.
33 Hall M: Mental capacity in the (civil) law: capacity, autonomy, and vulnerability. McGill Law Journal 2012;58:61–94.
34 Sherwin S: The Politics of Women's Health: Exploring Agency and Autonomy. Philadelphia, PA, Temple University Press, 1998.
35 Agich GJ: Dependence and Autonomy in Old Age: An Ethical Framework for Long-Term Care. Cambridge, Cambridge University Press, 2003.

Mary McNally
Faculties of Dentistry and Medicine, Dalhousie University
PO Box 15000, 5981 University Avenue
Halifax, NS B3H 4R2 (Canada)
E-Mail mary.mcnally@dal.ca

Theou O, Rockwood K (eds): Frailty in Aging. Biological, Clinical and Social Implications.
Interdiscipl Top Gerontol Geriatr. Basel, Karger, 2015, vol 41, pp 186–195 (DOI: 10.1159/000381236)

Frailty and Social Vulnerability

Melissa K. Andrew

Geriatric Medicine Research Unit, Dalhousie University, Halifax, N.S., Canada

Abstract

Both intrinsic and extrinsic factors contribute to health. Intrinsic factors are familiar topics in health research and include medical conditions, medications, genetics and frailty, while extrinsic factors stem from social and physical environments. This chapter builds on others in this volume, in which a deficit accumulation approach to frailty has been described. The concept of social vulnerability is presented. Social vulnerability stems from the accumulation of multiple and varied social problems and has bidirectional importance as a risk factor for poor health outcomes and as a pragmatic consideration for health care provision and planning. Importantly, the social factors that contribute to overall social vulnerability come into play at different levels of influence (individual, family and friends, peer groups, institutions and society at large). A social ecology perspective is discussed as a useful framework for considering social vulnerability, as it allows for attention to each of these levels of influence. Tying together what we currently understand about frailty (in medical and basic science models) and social vulnerability, the scaling potential of deficit accumulation is discussed, given that deficit accumulation can be understood to occur at many levels, from the (sub-)cellular level to tissues, organisms/complex systems and societies.

Many factors contribute to health; this concept will no doubt be abundantly clear to readers of this book. In order to make sense of such masses of influences, it is useful to consider the distinction between *intrinsic* and *extrinsic* contributors to health. Intrinsic factors include such considerations as medical conditions, medications, genetics and frailty itself, representing impaired repair mechanisms. Extrinsic contributors are factors external to an individual, stemming from social and physical environments. Some factors are in a gray area, with relevance to both categories. For example, socioeconomic (extrinsic) factors contribute to smoking and dietary intake, both of which might be construed as intrinsic contributors to health. Nevertheless, the distinction is a useful one to make and allows study of the role of how each realm is important for health and health outcomes.

It is noncontroversial that health has important social determinants. These include socioeconomic status (SES) (e.g. educational attainment, occupation, income and wealth or deprivation); social relationships and support from family and friends (which can be instrumental, as in hands-on help, or emotional) [1, 2]; engagement in group activities in one's community [3, 4]; mastery (feelings of control over life circumstances) [5]; and contextual factors relating to our neighborhoods, communities and societies [6, 7]. Some of these factors are relevant on the individual level, while others relate to connections between people and are thus properties of the relationships themselves. One particularity of the literature on social factors that might be relevant to health is that it is situated in a number of distinct disciplines and academic traditions. The terminology can thus be confusing; encountering similar terms may give a false sense of common ground when, in fact, different things are meant, and different terms may be used to represent what is in fact the same concept [8].

Traditionally, each social factor is studied 'one at a time', which has the benefit of keeping things simple and attributing (supposedly) 'independent' influence to each variable on its own. Studies show, for example, that living alone is associated with worse health outcomes; that volunteering is great for one's health; and that people who live in a neighborhood with low rates of crime, graffiti, and higher levels of trust (e.g. no 'pay before you pump' rules at the gas station) enjoy better health [9–11]. However, social circumstances are undoubtedly complex, and such 'one at a time' models, even when adjusting for confounding variables using statistical methods, run the risk of misclassifying risk and missing the point. Consider two older women who live alone. One is very isolated, rarely leaving home and receiving no regular visitors. Were she to become ill or fall, she might not be found for days. The other, although she lives alone, regularly socializes with a wide network of friends and family and engages in regular activities outside the home. If something were to happen to her, someone would notice much more quickly. Thus, although these two women both live alone and may be alike in many of the ways that research studies might usually take into account (age, health status, and even SES for the sake of argument), their social circumstances are very different.

Another way to think about social circumstances in relation to health is by using the concept of *social vulnerability* (SV) and the related idea of *social reserve*. SV captures the degree to which a person's overall social situation leaves him or her susceptible to further insults (either health-related or social). Considered as the inverse, social reserve is the degree of resilience that a well-connected and supportive social situation might impart. Ideally, capturing SV in an inclusive way serves to unify different domains of social factors that might influence health while capturing a holistic picture of the social factors that are at play for a given individual.

Social Vulnerability and Its Measurement

How can multiple social variables, with different levels of influence (on the individual-to-group continuum) be taken into account all at once? Here, a deficit accumulation approach provides a useful way forward. SV can be operationalized and measured as an index of social problems, or 'deficits', such that the more social deficits one has, the more vulnerability to adverse outcomes one has. Viewed in this way, the Social Vulnerability Index (SVI) approach is akin to the frailty index, which has been introduced earlier in this volume. Social variables representing many different domains are included (e.g. SES, living situation, social supports, social engagement, and neighborhood context); for a maximally holistic view, even domains that are traditionally viewed as part of other disciplines can be considered, such as socially relevant functional abilities (here, we can think of telephone use and the ability to mobilize outside one's home) and psychological characteristics (including a sense of mastery or control over one's circumstances and self-efficacy or self-esteem). Each variable is coded such that absence of the potential deficit is given a 0 (e.g. lives with others) and presence of the deficit is a 1 (e.g. lives alone). Intermediate values can be applied for ordered response categories, such as frequent social engagement at least once per week (0), occasional social engagement (0.5), and no social engagement (1). Points are summed across variables, and the total is divided by the total number of variables considered. For example, a person who has 3 of 30 social deficits would have SVI = 0.1, and someone with 12 of 30 would have SVI = 0.4 [12].

Experience with the SVI to date has shown that SV tends to increase with age [12]. Interestingly, despite this average tendency, aging does not just bring an inevitable march toward worsening social circumstances; there is also room for stabilization and even improvement. While we tend to think of women as being more socially connected than men, women have higher levels of SV on average [12]. The reasons for this are not clear, but analysis of the domains that contribute to SV suggests that women are most vulnerable in their living situation and in widowhood, even though they greatly compensate with stronger ties to friends and the broader community [13]. Notably, whereas the frailty index commonly records a 'zero state' (defined as the absence of any of the defining physical, functional or health deficits), in studies to date, no one has had zero SV [12, 14].

Outcomes of Social Vulnerability

SV predicts health outcomes, independent of age, sex and frailty. For example, SV has been associated with increased cognitive decline (measured as a clinically meaningful decline in cognitive test performance), with each additional social deficit being associated with a 3% increased odds of cognitive decline. Dividing a group into three SVI levels (high, medium and low), individuals with high SV had a 36% increased odds of experiencing cognitive decline compared with those with low SV [15]. Increasing SV was associated with a greater risk of mortality in two independent samples of older Canadians. For each additional social deficit contributing to overall SV, mortality increased by 5–8%. This study also identified a meaningful survival gradient across the levels of SV [12]. Perhaps most strikingly, considering only older people with no evident health deficits (those whose frailty index scores equaled zero), older people with high SV had 2.5 times the risk of five-year mortality, representing an absolute increase in mortality of 20% [14].

Context Matters

Given the broad definition of social circumstances and contributors to SV, it stands to reason that context, or the neighborhoods and societies in which we live, matters. One way to examine this potential effect is to compare neighborhoods and communities within the same country, such as by postal code linkage to census data and aggregate measures of neighborhood SES or deprivation. Doing so has contributed to the social ecology model of SV presented here. For example, in the English Longitudinal Study on Ageing, frailty was associated with neighborhood deprivation, such that people living in more deprived neighborhoods had higher levels of frailty on average, independent of individual SES [16]. Notably, as in so many other studies of social determinants of health, this was a gradient effect, rather than a threshold effect: it did not just apply to those in the poorest neighborhoods or to the most frail. Replication across countries, with attention to relevant differences in social conditions, is another means of taking context into account. The association between SV and mortality has also been replicated in the Survey of Health, Ageing and Retirement in Europe (SHARE), with interesting differences identified according to the social welfare model; SV predicted mortality in the Mediterranean and Continental welfare models, but not in the Nordic welfare model [17]. Another analysis of SHARE found that average levels of frailty across Europe were correlated with national economic indicators, such as gross domestic product [18].

Clinical Relevance of Social Vulnerability

SV has dual (and bidirectional) relevance to clinical care; in the first instance, as outlined above, it is a risk factor for poor outcomes. Pragmatically, social circumstances also have important consequences for planning home supports for frail older people and for discharge planning to facilitate the transition from hospital to home. Consideration of social circumstances, including living situation, marital status, education and occupational background, the presence of caregivers, caregiver strain and burnout, housing type and accessibility, the availability of formal home supports, and whether there is a 'care gap' or need for further supports, is integral to comprehensive geriatric assessment and key to care planning [19].

The ecological framework approach to SV can also be used to inform clinicians in cases of 'social admissions' or social presentations to acute care. Social admissions are unfortunately often viewed in derogatory terms, with terminology in the literature varying from 'acopia' (nominally from the Latin, as in *absence of coping*) to 'bed-blocker', 'GOMER' ('Get Out of My Emergency Room'), and 'home care impossible' [20–22]. Although the existing literature is limited, these are vulnerable patients with high rates of poor outcomes who deserve a careful and considerate workup and approach. For example, one UK study found that a diagnosis of 'acopia' was associated with high levels of frailty and a 22% in-hospital mortality rate; this finding highlights both problems with professionalism when value judgments are assigned to patients (as in, 'she is only a social admission') and poor diagnostic perspicuity. Underlying medical contributions were frequently present; only 6% of patients so labeled actually had no acute medical issues identified after a proper workup [23]. Among 253 patients in a Swiss study of patients triaged in the emergency department as 'home care impossible', 'undertriaging' (assigning patients with nonspecific symptoms to lower-acuity triage categories than their actual condition would warrant) was identified in 26% of cases, and acute medical problems were eventually identified in 51% [21]. This points to a broader problem of frail older adults being undertriaged in emergency department settings when presenting symptoms are not recognized as signals of underlying serious illness [24].

Often, then, what seems to be a 'social problem' on the surface has underlying acute and serious medical causes that will be missed without a proper workup. In addition, social factors are themselves complex. A structured approach to this complexity and to the multiple levels of influence by which social factors can act is key to providing good clinical care. A social ecology framework provides a useful approach to considering potential contributing social factors at each of the levels of the multiple nested spheres of influence (fig. 1). Consideration should be given to *patient factors* (e.g. unrecognized illness; pain; cognitive decline; behavioral and psychological symptoms of dementia; psychiatric conditions; polypharmacy), *family and informal caregiver factors* (e.g. caregiver stress, safety, financial considerations, the home living environment, a lack of a viable 'back-up plan' in case the caregiver becomes ill or is unavailable), *peer group factors* (e.g. formal or informal engagement or lack thereof in community social activities), *institutional factors* (e.g. the availability of home care services, respite care or other home supports that may or may not match care requirements), and *societal and policy factors* (e.g. government policies to support caregivers, the presence of a generally supportive and socially cohesive community, the accessibility and suitability of the built environment and to the age-friendliness of communities).

The Scaling Problem

Generally speaking, the deficit accumulation approach has a number of advantages. It allows simultaneous consideration of a large number of variables that may or may not individually influence health but that may be important when taken as a whole. It

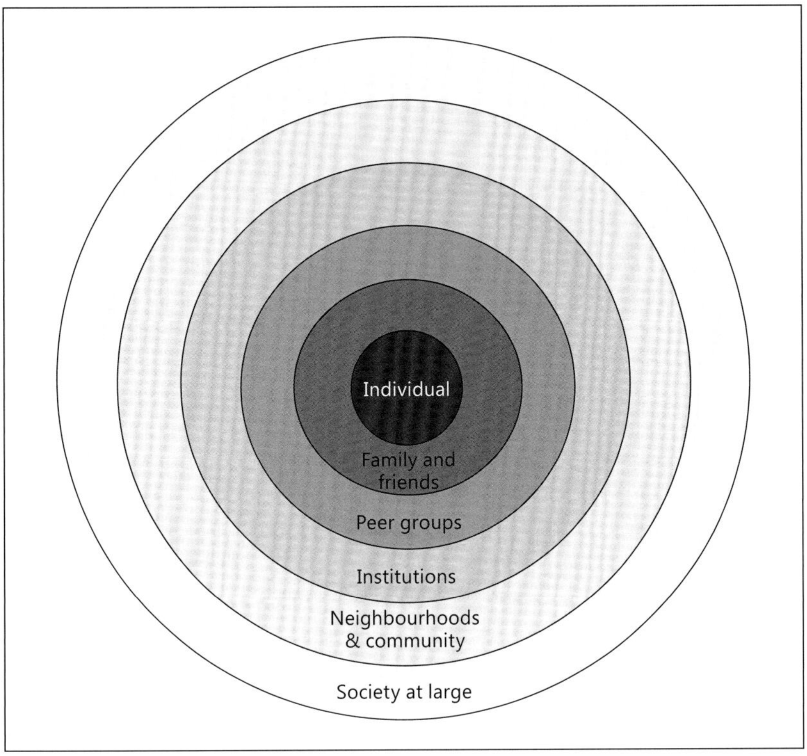

Fig. 1. Individuals are embedded in a nested social structure; a social ecology perspective provides a framework for considering social influences at each level. Adapted from [13].

also avoids problems that can be encountered in traditional statistical models regarding assumptions of parameter independence in the absence of multiple collinearity. Index variables allow us to capture a graded continuum of risk, rather than collapsing risk into an arbitrary number of risk categories [12]. Specific to the consideration of SV, an advantage of a deficit accumulation approach is that it allows consideration of numerous social factors from multiple domains (e.g. living situation, social supports, social engagement, mastery, SES). As outlined above for the example of social admissions to the hospital, a social ecology framework allows us to consider which aspects of SV are active at various levels of influence and also how interventions might be targeted at important elements or domains of SV.

Another great advantage of a deficit accumulation approach, which is attractive on both theoretical and practical levels, is scaling. Readers will have seen examples of deficit accumulation at the sub-cellular level earlier in this book. Deficits can also accumulate at the tissue level and at the level of systems (as with individual people or animals, which are effectively complex systems). Of particular relevance to the present discussion, deficits can also accumulate at levels higher than individuals, or at the social level, pertaining to social environments and circumstances (fig. 2).

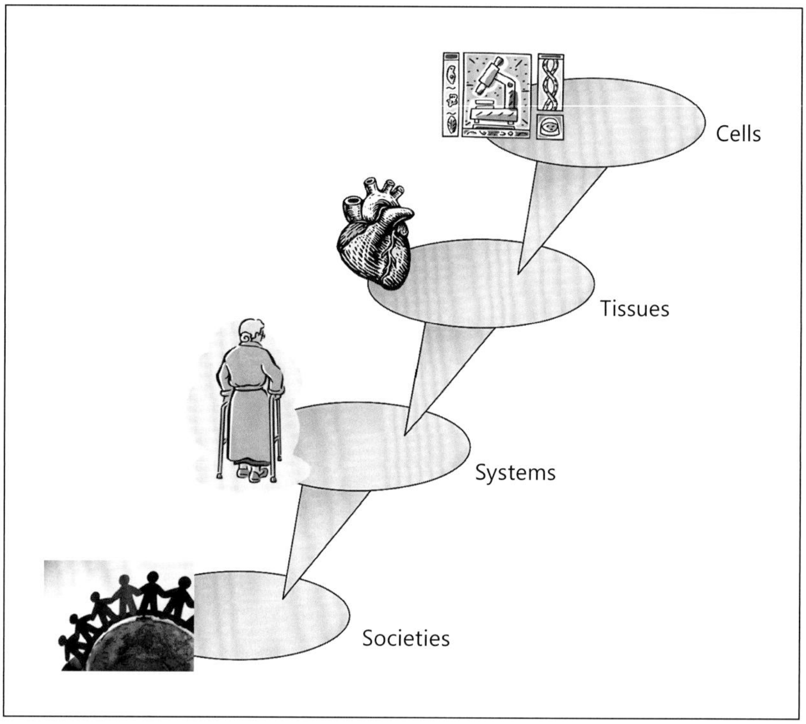

Fig. 2. Deficit accumulation can be scaled from the (sub-)cellular level to tissues, complex systems or organisms and societies as a whole.

Questions That Remain

Is Deficit Accumulation a One-Way Street?

Deficits accumulate as people age, and as these deficits accumulate, people become more frail and thus more prone to adverse outcomes. However, it is likely that *bad* things (deficits) may not be the only things that accrue (or indeed stay static or improve) with aging. It is possible to see that *protective* assets may also accumulate, stay static, or decline with age. One key methodological and conceptual question that remains is this: is the presence of an asset the same as the absence of a deficit? It seems intuitive that having assets and not having deficits is not the same thing; for example, being in a supportive relationship isn't the same as not suffering domestic abuse. While the deficit accumulation model has allowed us to capture a gradient of SV, a model that also allows for explicit consideration of assets may improve the descriptive utility. This would allow us to address such questions as 'Might having assets cancel out having deficits?' (this has been seen, for example, in the case of education and midlife exercise cancelling out, at least in part, the increased risk of late-life dementia of the ApoE4 haplotype) [25, 26]. Recent attempts to add a 'protection index' to the Frailty Index are of interest [27]. The choice of items as 'external' protection (education, exercise) overlaps with SV, leaving open the question of whether these are best coded as assets or deficits. Another key question will be to investigate *transitions* in health using models that allow for improvement as well as for decline.

Queuing Theory and Accumulation

Deficit accumulation is a balance between arrival (or challenge) and wait time (time taken to be processed or repaired). In the mathematical modeling of frailty and reserve, we can usefully apply queuing theory. Queuing theory aims to describe systems in which items (e.g. people lining up in a shop) accumulate in a queue. It is based on Little's law, which states that the average number of items in a queuing system *(L)* equals the average arrival rate (λ) multiplied by the average waiting time of an item in the system, or *W*. This can be expressed as $L = \lambda W$ [28, 29]. Queuing theory has been applied in many diverse fields, from communications systems (wait times in telephone call center service queues may be an example that we all love to hate) to computer architecture and organizational management.

Recently, Mitnitski et al. have reformulated Little's law so that *L* equals the number of deficits accumulated, λ is the stresses or challenges to the system (which can be intrinsic or extrinsic) and *W* is the recovery time (the time taken to 'process' or deal with the challenge so that it does not 'stick' to become a lasting contribution to the number of deficits *L*) [30]. When processing or recovery times are fast, most people will have few (or no) deficits; this is what we observe at younger ages. As recovery times slow, the distribution will gradually shift in favor of the accumulation of deficits (which will happen in an age-related fashion as recovery time lengthens). Recovery time is therefore proportional to the average number of deficits that an individual possesses. Average recovery time increases with age, even if we assume a constant intensity of the 'arrival' or of stressors or deficits in the environment (both intrinsic and extrinsic). Recovery time thus becomes the key factor to understand. Based on prior analyses, recovery time seems to increase exponentially with age, along with the observed number of deficits that 'stick' [30]. As recovery time lengthens, it is harder to process, clear or deflect deficits, and they will tend to accumulate; this is indeed what we observe (on average) with aging.

Why does recovery time lengthen with age? This may have to do with various mechanisms on a whole spectrum from biochemical (e.g. repair mechanisms for DNA and chromosomal damage) to cellular and tissue changes (e.g. elasticity of cell fibers and electrical conductivity potentials); factors relating to immunity, inflammation and hormonal axis factors; and also organ system influences (e.g. loss of redundancy as cells die or become less functional; at the tissue level, we have many more nephrons than we need until too many are damaged, in which case kidney dysfunction develops) [31]. Importantly, extrinsic factors such as the social environments in which people live are also likely to impact both the arrival of deficits in the queue and the organism's recovery time and capabilities; this is an important area for further enquiry.

What to Do About Social Vulnerability: Clinical and Policy Applications

Identifying the problem will take us only so far. There is clearly a great need to be able to understand the importance of SV for health care and care planning and to be able to intervene to improve people's circumstances and their health. We must move toward a clearer understanding of SV and its assessment in clinical care settings. Formalizing clinical approaches to SV is clearly an area for further work.

A structured approach to SV and its contributors, such as the social ecology framework discussed above, presents a way forward for considering potential interventions at each level of influence. This includes addressing *patient factors* (e.g. improving educational opportunities across the life course, assisting with access to available pension and insurance supports, identifying and managing contributing medical issues), *family and informal caregiver factors* (e.g. supporting caregivers to minimize stress, providing supports in the home living environment), *peer group factors* (e.g. creating opportunities for both formal and informal engagement in the broader community, such as by supporting programming for older adults by community groups and providing accessible transportation options and common space in communal living facilities), *institutional factors* (e.g. policy support for accessible and comprehensive home care services and respite care), and *societal and policy factors* (e.g. government policies to support caregivers, attention to accessibility in the built environment and to the age-friendliness of communities) [19].

Understanding how deficits accumulate and scale from cells to tissues, systems and societies presents us with both a fascinating scientific challenge and a way forward for considering the complexities of health, health care and social care. Much is known, but there is clearly more work to be done.

References

1 Holt-Lunstad J, Smith TB, Layton JB: Social relationships and mortality risk: a meta-analytic review. PLoS Med 2010;7:e1000316.

2 Berkman LF: Social support, social networks, social cohesion and health. Soc Work Health Care 2000;31:3–14.

3 Bennett KM: Social engagement as a longitudinal predictor of objective and subjective health. Eur J Ageing 2005;2:48–55.

4 Krueger KR, Wilson RS, Kamenetsky JM, Barnes LL, Bienias JL, Bennett DA: Social engagement and cognitive function in old age. Exp Aging Res 2009;35:45–60.

5 Marmot M: Status Syndrome: How Your Social Standing Directly Affects Your Health and Life Expectancy. London, Bloomsbury Publishing, 2004.

6 Subramanian SV, Kim DJ, Kawachi I: Social trust and self-rated health in US communities: a multilevel analysis. J Urban Health 2002;79(4 suppl 1):S21–S34.

7 Putnam RD: Bowling Alone: The Collapse and Revival of American Community. New York, Simon & Schuster, 2000.

8 Andrew MK: Le capital social et la santé des personnes âgées. Retraite et Société 2005;46:129–143.

9 Lochner KA, Kawachi I, Brennan RT, Buka SL: Social capital and neighborhood mortality rates in Chicago. Soc Sci Med 2003;56:1797–1805.

10 Barron JS, Tan EJ, Yu Q, Song M, McGill S, Fried LP: Potential for intensive volunteering to promote the health of older adults in fair health. J Urban Health 2009;86:641–653.

11 Gill T, Taylor AW, Pengelly A: A population-based survey of factors relating to the prevalence of falls in older people. Gerontology 2005;51:340–345.

12 Andrew MK, Mitnitski A, Rockwood K: Social vulnerability, frailty, and mortality in elderly people. PLoS One 2008;3:e2232.

13 Andrew M, Keefe J: Social vulnerability from a social ecology perspective: a cohort study of older adults from the National Population Health Survey of Canada. BMC Geriatr 2014;14:90.
14 Andrew M, Mitnitski A, Kirkland SA, Rockwood K: The impact of social vulnerability on the survival of the fittest older adults. Age Ageing 2012;41:161–165.
15 Andrew MK, Rockwood K: Social vulnerability predicts cognitive decline in a prospective cohort of older Canadians. Alzheimers Dement 2010;6:319–325.
16 Lang IA, Hubbard RE, Andrew MK, Llewellyn DJ, Melzer D, Rockwood K: Neighborhood deprivation, individual socioeconomic status, and frailty in older adults. J Am Geriatr Soc 2009;57:1776–1780.
17 Wallace L, Theou O, Pena F, Rockwood K, Andrew MK: Social vulnerability as a predictor of mortality and disability: cross-country differences in the Survey of Health, Aging, and Retirement in Europe (SHARE). Aging Clin Exp Res DOI: 10.1007/s40520-014-0271-6.
18 Theou O, Brothers TD, Rockwood MR, Haardt D, Mitnitski A, Rockwood K: Exploring the relationship between national economic indicators and relative fitness and frailty in middle-aged and older Europeans. Age Ageing 2013;42:614–619.
19 Andrew MK, Powell C: An approach to 'the social admission'. Can J General Internal Medicine 2014; in press.
20 Oliver D: 'Acopia' and 'social admission' are not diagnoses: why older people deserve better. J R Soc Med 2008;101:168–174.
21 Rutschmann OT, Chevalley T, Zumwald C, Luthy C, Vermeulen B, Sarasin FP: Pitfalls in the emergency department triage of frail elderly patients without specific complaints. Swiss Med Wkly 2005;135:145–150.
22 Shem S: The House of God. New York, Richard Marek Publishers, 1978.
23 Kee YY, Rippingale C: The prevalence and characteristic of patients with 'acopia'. Age Ageing 2009;38: 103–105.
24 Goldstein JP, Andrew MK, Travers A: Frailty in older adults using pre-hospital care and the emergency department: a narrative review. Can Geriatr J 2012; 15:16–22.
25 Wang HX, Gustafson DR, Kivipelto M, Pedersen NL, Skoog I, Windblad B, Fratiglioni L: Education halves the risk of dementia due to apolipoprotein epsilon4 allele: a collaborative study from the Swedish brain power initiative. Neurobiol Aging 2012;33:1007.e1–e7.
26 Rovio S, Kareholt I, Helkala EL, Viitanen M, Winblad B, Tuomilehto J, Soininen H, Nissinen A, Kivipelto M: Leisure-time physical activity at midlife and the risk of dementia and Alzheimer's disease. Lancet Neurol 2005;4:705–711.
27 Wang C, Song X, Mitnitski A, Fang X, Tang Z, Yu P, Rockwood K: Effect of health protective factors on health deficit accumulation and mortality risk in older adults in the Beijing Longitudinal Study of Aging. J Am Geriatr Soc 2014;62:821–828.
28 Little JDC: A proof for the queuing formula: L=λ W. Operation Research 1961;59:383–387.
29 Little JDC: Little's law as viewed on its 50th anniversary. Operation Research 2011;59:536–549.
30 Mitnitski A, Song X, Rockwood K: Assessing biological aging: the origin of deficit accumulation. Biogerontology 2013;16:709–717.
31 Lopez-Otin C, Blasco MA, Partridge L, Serrano M, Kroemer G: The hallmarks of aging. Cell 2013;153: 1194–1217.

Melissa K. Andrew
c/o Division of Geriatric Medicine
Veterans' Memorial Building, 5955 Veterans' Memorial Lane
Halifax, NS, B3H 2E1 (Canada)
E-Mail mandrew@dal.ca

Author Index

Subject Index